GROCERY SHOPPING GUIDE

3rd Edition

**A Consumer's Manual
for Selecting Foods Low
Dietary Fat, Saturated Fat**

Nelda Mercer, M.S., R.
Assistant Director of Pr
MedSport Cardiac Prog

Carl Orringer, M.D.
Director of Preventive Cardiology
and Cardiac Rehabilitation Programs
University of Michigan Medical Center

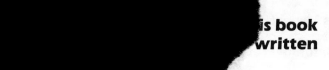

is book written

As a health care facility, the University of Michigan Medical Center has a strong commitment to wellness — not just the health of our patients, but that of the whole community.

To promote nutritional wellness, our dietary and medical experts at MedSport have developed the *Grocery Shopping Guide* to help you make wise nutritional buys.

Initially, the *Guide* was developed as an educational service for U of M MedSport patients who suffered from heart disease, high cholesterol and high blood pressure. We soon realized that *everyone* could benefit from the knowledge contained in this *Guide,* and are now pleased to offer it to the general public.

Some of the most important steps you can take towards healthier eating habits are those taken behind the grocery cart. The *Grocery Shopping Guide* is a comprehensive and convenient "map" guiding you to the best nutritional choices for you and your family.

Bon appetit, and good shopping!

Special Note:
The information contained in this book is correct as of the time this book was prepared for publication. However, since ingredients or processing may change from time to time, it is essential that you continue to read ingredient labels to determine how appropriate the food choices are. The criteria presented for each food classification will enable you to evaluate new and/or additional food products that were not included.

Acknowledgements

The authors wish to express their sincere appreciation to John Forsyth, Executive Director, University of Michigan Hospitals, for his enthusiastic support of this book.

The authors also wish to recognize the direction and help given by LaVaughn Palma-Davis, M.A., Administrative Director of U of M MedSport, in getting this book launched.

We are especially grateful to Kathy Sadd Quinn, M.S., R.D. and Elizabeth Burt, R.N., I.A.C.P. certified, for their tireless proofing and attention to detail throughout all stages of this book. The contributions by Terry Knox, R.D., and Diane Hurst, R.D., were invaluable as they spent many devoted hours in the grocery store aisles reviewing food products. We are also grateful to Kathy Rhodes, Ph.D., R.D. and Lisa Bookstein, M.S., R.D. for their expert review of the nutritional text and final proofing of the book.

We also wish to recognize the work of Linda Wicklund, M.S., R.D., Sue Valiquett, M.S., R.D., Patricia L. Weise, R.D., and dietetic students Donna Davis and Donna Donakowski who worked on previous editions.

We are particularly grateful to Steven Riddle, M.S. and David Trumbull for their technical assistance in formatting the original document, and to Douglas H. Okamoto for his accuracy and persistence on the computer while entering and reformatting this revised edition.

Finally, the authors wish to say a very special thank you to our friends and co-workers at MedSport, who in one way or another were involved with all stages of this book.

CONTENTS

Food Products, continued

INTRODUCTION

Heart disease is the number one cause of death and disability in the United States. At least half of all American deaths are due to heart attacks (approximately one per minute). Did you know that a powerful means of preventing heart disease is in your grocery store? You first have to know how to find it! The purpose of the *Grocery Shopping Guide* is to assist you in making wise food selections which are appropriate for controlling the intake of total fat, saturated fat, cholesterol, sodium and refined sugar, and increasing dietary fiber.

Scientific studies have shown that diets high in saturated fat and cholesterol adversely affect health by predisposing people to heart disease, obesity and certain types of cancer.[1] On the other hand, it has been shown that diets *lower* in fat and *high* in dietary fiber reduce blood cholesterol and blood pressure, lower elevated blood sugar levels in persons with diabetes, and improve health and well-being.[2]

Our goal is to teach you to make better food choices so that you can prevent or decrease your risk for heart disease. We recognize that while no guidelines can guarantee health or well-being, good eating habits based on wise food selection can help you stay healthy and may even improve your health.

The *Grocery Shopping* Guide is an aisle-by-aisle listing of foods by brand name, designating those that are acceptable and those that are not recommended based on their total fat and saturated fat content. Foods that are high in sodium, as well as those that are good sources of dietary fiber are identified. Although the cholesterol content of food is not specified, food products containing egg yolks, which are a major source of cholesterol, are identified with the symbol (●).

UNDERSTANDING THE BASICS

Why is it important to read food labels?

What is ingredient labeling?

Since more than half of the foods we eat are packaged and processed, learning to read and understand labels is a critical part of analyzing and improving our diets. Many processed foods contain large amounts of saturated fats, cholesterol, sugar and sodium. By reading the labels of processed foods, you can determine which products are healthful.

Packaged foods must list ingredients on the label. Ingredients are listed in order of concentration in the product: largest quantity (first), down to the smallest quantity (last).

The only foods not required to list all ingredients are so-called standardized foods. Standards of identity, set by the Food and Drug Administration (FDA), require foods called by a particular name (such as catsup or mayonnaise) to contain certain mandatory ingredients. These mandatory ingredients in standardized foods need not be listed on the label. Manufacturers may add optional ingredients, but these must be listed on the label.

All products containing fat must list the kind of vegetable or animal fat used.

What is nutrition labeling?

The following is a brief discussion of nutrition labeling as it exists today but will soon be phased out with the new labeling reform described below. Federal law currently requires that nutritional information be listed on certain products. These include all enriched or fortified foods and all foods for which a nutritional claim is made. Nutrition labels must contain the following information:

1. Serving (portion) size: the amount of food for which nutrition information is given, such as one slice, three ounces, one-half cup.

2. The amount of food energy (in calories); the amount of protein, fat and carbohydrate (in grams) contained in one serving.

3. Percentages of the U.S. Recommended Daily Allowances (USRDA) for protein, vitamin A, vitamin C, the B vitamins (thiamin, niacin, riboflavin), calcium and iron.

Nutrition Labeling Reform:

The 1990s will be the decade of sweeping reform in nutrition labeling. In the fall of 1989 the Committee on Nutrition Components of Food Labeling, Food and Nutrition Board, Institute of Medicine, National Academy of Science[3] issued recommendations for labeling reform. The committee's overall goal was to redesign food labels so that they provide nutrient information that can aid consumers in adopting or adhering to healthy diets. These proposals were passed by the House of Representatives in July, 1990, and by the Senate in late October, 1990. On November 9, 1990, President Bush signed into law the Nutrition Labeling and Education Act of 1990 (Pub. L. 101-535). Under the new law the following changes will be mandated by the FDA:

1. Mandatory nutrition labeling will be required on all food and beverages (with few exceptions).

2. Standardized serving sizes will be established for 159 food

product categories to assure reasonable and uniform serving size upon which consumers can make nutrition comparisons among food products.

3. Nutritional labeling must now include values for the following nutrients based on pre-established standardized serving sizes: total calories, total calories derived from fat, amount of total fat, saturated fat, cholesterol, sodium, carbohydrates, sugars, dietary fiber, and protein.

4. The current U.S. Recommended Dietary Allowances (USRDAs) will be replaced with Reference Daily Intakes (RDIs) for protein and 26 vitamins and minerals, and Daily Reference Values (DRVs) for eight food components considered important to maintenance of good health (i.e. fat, saturated fatty acids, unsaturated fatty acids, cholesterol, carbohydrate, fiber, sodium and potassium). RDIs and DRVs are designed to help consumers interpret information about the amount of a nutrient present in a food and to compare the nutritional values of foods.

5. The new labeling laws will also establish quantitative definitions for descriptive terms such as "low", "reduced" and "free." For example, a tentative final rule has been issued defining cholesterol descriptions as follows:

- A food labeled "cholesterol free" must contain less than 2 mg. cholesterol per serving, with 5 grams or less total fat ($\leqslant$20% fat, dry wt.) and 2 grams or less saturated fat ($\leqslant$6% saturated fat, dry wt.).
- A food labeled "low cholesterol" must contain 20 mg. cholesterol or less per serving, with 5 grams or less total fat ($\leqslant$20% fat, dry wt.) and 2 grams or less saturated fat (6% saturated fat, dry wt.).
- A food labeled "reduced cholesterol" must contain at least 75% less cholesterol compared with the level in the food it replaces,

accompanied by an explanatory statement of comparison (e.g., cholesterol content has been reduced from 100 mg. to 25 mg. per serving).

Definitions for "lite" and "light" will also be established as well as for phrases such as "good source of," "significant source of" and "excellent source of." For a comprehensive listing of existing working policy definitions of other descriptors, see appendix A, page 358-362.

The new law also preempts state labeling laws (with exception of safety warning labels) which are not consistent with federal requirements. Manufacturers will be given two years in which to comply with the newly established food labeling laws. Consumers will most likely start to notice these changes within the coming year. Our next edition of the *Guide* will contain a more detailed description of these changes along with guidelines on how to interpret this information.

What is cholesterol and how does it affect my health?

Cholesterol is a waxy substance used by the body to manufacture: (1) certain hormones which control the body's metabolism, (2) bile acids which aid in fat digestion, and (3) cell membranes, the outer boundaries of each cell of the body, which help to maintain the delicate chemical balance required for normal bodily functions. Although cholesterol is essential for life, our bodies produce sufficient quantities to meet our physiological needs. In other words, if we never ate a single milligram of cholesterol we would not suffer from a deficiency!

There are two types of cholesterol:

Dietary cholesterol is cholesterol that is in the food you eat. It is present only in foods of animal origin (e.g., meat, poultry, fish, dairy products), *not* in foods of plant origin (e.g., vegetables, vegetable oil, fruits and grains). Dietary cholesterol, like saturated fat, tends to raise blood cholesterol. It has been estimated that dietary cholesterol raises serum cholesterol by 8-10 mg. per 100 mg. dietary cholesterol consumed per 1000 calories.[4,5]

Blood or serum cholesterol is cholesterol that is either manufactured in the liver or absorbed from the food you eat. It is carried in the blood for use by all parts of the body. Scientific studies have shown beyond doubt that high levels of cholesterol in the blood predispose individuals to the development of blockages in the blood vessels of the heart (coronary artery disease).[6,7]

Knowing your own cholesterol level is important. The National Cholesterol Education Program Expert Panel recently set guidelines for classifying blood cholesterol levels. They advise that a total cholesterol level less than 200 mg./dl. is desirable for adults over 20 years of age.[8] It has been shown that the risk of developing coronary artery disease steadily increases at cholesterol levels above 218 mg./dl.[9] The average blood cholesterol level for middle-aged men and women in the United States is about 215 mg./dl. The average cholesterol of a heart attack victim is 230-240 mg./dl.[10]

Certain diets have been shown to be effective in reducing blood cholesterol by as much as 10-30%.[11] Scientific studies have shown that for middle-aged men with cholesterol levels exceeding 250 mg./dl., every 1% reduction in blood cholesterol is associated with a 2% reduction in risk for a heart attack. Therefore, a sustained 10-30% reduction of cholesterol represents a 20-60% reduction in heart attack risk.[12]

What is HDL and LDL cholesterol?

You may have heard about the different types of blood cholesterol and their effect in determining your risk for coronary artery disease.

Since fat and cholesterol do not dissolve in blood, in order for them to be transported in the bloodstream, they must be carried by specialized transport proteins. These packages of fat and protein are called lipoproteins. Lipoproteins are classified according to their density.

High-density lipoproteins (HDL): Lipoproteins that contain a small amount of cholesterol and carry cholesterol away from the heart and coronary arteries to the liver for reprocessing or removal from the body are called high-density lipoproteins.

Researchers have noted that persons with higher levels of HDL have a lower incidence of heart disease.[13,14] Therefore, HDLs have been known as the "good" cholesterol. Most persons in industrialized countries with low levels of HDL (less than 35 mg./dl.) are at higher risk for developing coronary heart disease. A well-known exception to this rule occurs in certain populations of vegetarians who tend to have low levels of all categories of lipoproteins, and have a very low risk of developing coronary heart disease.[15,16] While the benefits of having a high level of HDL cholesterol in free living North Americans are well known, the only group of persons who have clearly been demonstrated to benefit from efforts directed at raising levels of HDL cholesterol is middle-aged men who have low levels of HDL cholesterol, and elevated levels of LDL cholesterol and triglycerides.[17] Thus, it has not been established with certainty that raising HDL cholesterol levels inevitably lowers coronary heart disease risk.

Low density lipoproteins (LDL): Lipoproteins that contain the greatest amounts of cholesterol and are responsible for carrying cholesterol to the cells of the body are called low-density lipoproteins. When cholesterol-rich LDL is present in excess, this cholesterol may become deposited in the walls of arteries, initiating the disease known as atherosclerosis (hardening of the arteries). For this reason, LDL is sometimes called "bad" cholesterol. High levels of LDL are therefore associated with an increased risk of coronary heart disease. A "desirable" level of LDL cholesterol in adults depends upon the number of risk factors a person has for coronary heart disease. These risk factors include the male sex, a family history of coronary heart disease in a parent or sibling under 55 years of age, cigarette smoking of $1/2$ pack (10 cigarettes) or more per day, high blood pressure, diabetes mellitus, low levels of HDL cholesterol (<35 mg./dl.), a history of stroke or impaired blood flow to the legs and a body weight of greater than 30% above one's ideal weight. If a person has two or more of these risk factors, or if he or she has already been found to have coronary heart disease, the goal for LDL cholesterol levels should be less than 130 mg./dl. For those persons with zero or one risk factor and no coronary heart disease, the goal should be less than 160 mg./dl.[8]

How does diet affect blood cholesterol?

It is important to understand that three factors increase blood cholesterol: (1) eating too much cholesterol; (2) eating too much saturated fat; and (3) eating an excess of calories, resulting in obesity.[18] In the typical American diet, the **saturated fat** content is the strongest contributor to raising blood cholesterol.[19] Excess calories and cholesterol in foods also contribute, but to a lesser extent. Therefore, in addition to decreasing dietary cholesterol intake to less than 300 mg. per day and consuming appropriate calories to maintain desirable weight, it is probably even more important to decrease saturated fat to 10% or less of total daily calories. Identifying foods that are high in saturated fat is not as easy as identifying those foods that are high in cholesterol. Food labels may also be confusing and misleading. For example, some foods may be labeled "No Cholesterol" yet contain high levels of saturated fats which contribute to elevating blood cholesterol! A major emphasis of this *Grocery Shopping Guide* is to identify foods high in **saturated fats** so that you can avoid or limit their use.

How do fats affect cholesterol?

Fats are the major class of foods that affect cholesterol levels. Some fat will increase the blood cholesterol levels, while others can decrease the levels.

Dietary fats are a mixture of three major types: saturated, monounsaturated and polyunsaturated. An understanding of this terminology is helpful in becoming familiar with the role of fat in the diet. Saturated, polyunsaturated and monounsaturated are all chemical terms. They refer to the structure and orientation of the molecules of carbon, hydrogen and oxygen.

What is saturated fat?

Saturated refers to a molecule which is filled with hydrogen atoms. It is saturated and will not accept any more hydrogen. An analogy would be to compare a saturated fat molecule to a household sponge. Once a sponge becomes "saturated" with water, it can no longer hold additional water. Below is a diagram of a *saturated* fat.

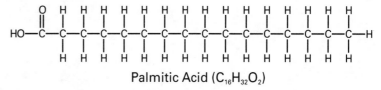

Palmitic Acid ($C_{16}H_{32}O_2$)

Saturated fats are solid at room temperature and play a major role in elevating blood cholesterol.[20] They are found predominantly in animal sources but can also be found in some vegetable sources:

Sources of Saturated Fats

Animal	Dairy Products	Plant
bacon and bacon fat	butter	cocoa butter (chocolate)
beef tallow	cheese	coconut oil
chicken fat	cream	palm kernel oil
lamb tallow	cream cheese	palm oil
lard	ice cream	vegetable shortening or hydrogenated oils made from any of the above
salt pork	sour cream	
	whole and 2% milk	

Nuts

coconut

What is monounsaturated fat?

When openings are created by a double bond between two carbons, the fat is not saturated. If one double bond (indicated by $=$) is present, the fat molecule is said to be monounsaturated. A *monounsaturated* fat is pictured below:

$$HO-C-C-C-C-C-C-C-C=C-C-C-C-C-C-C-C-C-H$$

Oleic Acid ($C_{18}H_{34}O_2$)

Monounsaturated fats are liquid at room temperature. When monounsaturated oils such as peanut or olive are stored in the refrigerator, they become solid; however, this does not make them saturated. Studies that were conducted in the 1950s and 1960s by Keys[4] and Hegstead[5] postulated that oleic acid (a monounsaturated fatty acid) is *neutral* in its effect on plasma cholesterol. In 1970 Keys[21] published a major epidemiological study that examined the associations among diet, plasma cholesterol, other risk factors and coronary heart disease (CHD) rates in several different populations within seven countries. This study demonstrated that CHD rates were low in the Mediterranean region where large quantities of olive oil are consumed. More recent clinical research studies,[22,23,24] have confirmed that monounsaturated fats (oleic acid) are equally as effective in lowering LDL cholesterol as are polyunsaturated fats, when substituted in the diet for saturated fats.

Monounsaturated fats are found primarily in vegetable oils, nuts and nut butters.

Sources of Monounsaturated Fats

Vegetable Oils

avocado oil
canola (low erucic acid
   rapeseed oil)
high oleic safflower oil
high oleic sunflower oil
olive oil
peanut oil

Vegetables/Fruits

avocados
olives

Nuts and Nut butters*

acorns
almonds
beechnuts
cashews
filberts or hazelnuts
hickory nuts
macadamia nuts
peanuts
pecans
pistachios

*The predominant fat in these nuts is monounsaturated.

What is polyunsaturated fat?

A fat with two or more double bonds is called polyunsaturated. This means there are four or more vacant spots that are not filled with hydrogen atoms. A *polyunsaturated* fat looks like this:

$$HO-C-C-C-C-C-C-C-C=C-C-C=C-C-C-C-C-C-H$$

Linoleic Acid ($C_{18}H_{32}O_2$)

Polyunsaturated fats are liquid at room temperature. These oils may become more viscous (thick) or cloudy when refrigerated but will still remain liquid. When replaced for saturated fats in the diet, polyunsaturated fats (like monounsaturated fats) lower LDL cholesterol.[20] Several potential drawbacks to consuming diets high in polyunsaturated fat exist. First of all, no large population group has ever consumed large quantities of polyunsaturated fatty acid with proven safety. Secondly, several research studies have shown that diets high in polyunsaturates may also lower protective HDL cholesterol levels.[25,26] On the other hand, a more recent study showed that HDL is not negatively affected if polyunsaturated fat consumption is kept to the current levels recommended by the National Cholesterol Education Program Step I diet (i.e., 30% or less total fat with 10% or less polyunsaturated fat).[27] Thirdly, it has been speculated that diets high in polyunsaturated fats result in the formation of oxidized LDL which is a type of LDL that is especially likely to cause plaque formation in blood vessels.[28] Further research to confirm this finding is necessary before firm conclusions can be drawn. Finally, a high intake of dietary polyunsaturated fat has also been shown to promote tumor growth in some laboratory animals fed low fat diets.[29] The applicability of this finding to humans remains uncertain.

Sources of Polyunsaturated Fats		
Vegetable Oils	**Nuts***	**Seeds**
safflower	Brazil nuts	sesame
sesame	butternuts	sunflower
sunflower	pine nuts	pumpkin
soybean	walnuts	
Other ■ Soft or liquid Margarines ■ Mayonnaise made from soybean or safflower oil		

*The predominant fat in these nuts is polyunsaturated.

Note: Although cottonseed oil is 52% polyunsaturated, it also contains 26% saturated fat (mostly palmitic acid which is known to elevate cholesterol). For this reason, it is not listed as a source of recommended polyunsaturated fat. However, cottonseed oil is an unsaturated oil and is therefore an acceptable fat ingredient in commercially prepared foods.

What about hydrogenated oils: are they good or bad fats?

Hydrogenation is a chemical process that changes liquid vegetable oil (unsaturated fat) to a more solid shortening (saturated fat) by adding hydrogen. The commercial food industry uses hydrogenated oils primarily in baked food products such as breads, crackers, cakes, cookies, etc. It is necessary to hydrogenate unsaturated oils in order to produce a desired texture and increase shelf life. Hydrogenated oils are more stable and resist oxidation which can cause rancidity and spoilage.

Hydrogenation primarily increases the amount of **monounsaturated** fatty acids and, to a lesser degree, increases the amount of saturated fatty acids (See Table 1). It is important to note that the biggest increase in saturated fat is in the form of stearic acid which has **not** been shown to cause an elevation in blood cholesterol levels in persons who already consume a low cholesterol diet.[30] Table 1 illustrates that as soybean oil becomes more hydrogenated, going from liquid to solid, the most significant change is that monounsaturated fat increases from 23 to 45 grams percent with a subsequent decrease in polyunsaturated fat from 58 to 26 grams percent. Scientists are unsure whether the monounsaturated fatty acids formed by hydrogenation are as beneficial as naturally occurring monounsaturated fatty acids. The reason for this uncertainty is that the process of hydrogenation causes the formation of *trans fatty* acids which in recent studies[31] have been shown to increase LDL cholesterol and decrease HDL cholesterol.

Table 1
Effect of Hydrogenation on Saturated Fat Content
(grams / 100 grams)

	Total Saturated	Stearic	Palmitic	Myristic	Mono	Poly
Soybean Oil	14	3.8	10.3	.1	23	58
Soybean Oil (hydrogenated)	15	5.0	9.8	.1	43	38
Tub Soybean Margarine	14	4.7	8.7	.1	37	27
Stick Soybean Margarine	13	4.9	8.1	.1	38	26
Soybean Shortening (soy/cottonseed)	25	10.6	14.1	.4	45	26
Change	+11	+6.8	+3.8	+.3	+22	−32
*Cottonseed Oil (non-hydrogenated)	**26**	2.3	**22.7**	.8	18	52

Source: United States Department of Agriculture, Agriculture Handbook No. 8-4: *Composition of Foods: Fats and Oils — Raw, Processed, and Prepared.* Washington, D.C., U.S. Government Printing Office, 1979.[32]

*Special Note: It is interesting to note that pure cottonseed oil (**non**-hydrogenated) is higher in total saturated fat (mostly from palmitic acid which is known to elevate cholesterol) than shortening produced from hydrogenated soybean/cottonseed oil blend. The authors conclude that cottonseed oil is the least preferred choice of all the unsaturated oils and should only be consumed in limited amounts.

In an effort to translate these scientific findings to practical applications for food selection, we present the following recommendations:

1. Limit **ALL** sources of fat, saturated as well as unsaturated.

2. Of the acceptable unsaturated fats, monounsaturates seem to be associated with the greatest health benefits. As a result, we recommend monounsaturated fat as the preferred choice.

3. Use sparingly those food products made with **hydrogenated** unsaturated oils such as canola, soybean, cottonseed, corn, safflower and sunflower. These hydrogenated oils are often found in margarines, shortenings, mayonnaise, salad dressings, and many commercially prepared baked goods.

4. Avoid hydrogenated oils or shortenings made from highly saturated oils such as coconut, palm and palm kernel. These oils contain high levels of lauric, myristic and palmitic acids which are known to elevate cholesterol.[20]

The following examples are of food labels listing **acceptable** shortenings from hydrogenated unsaturated oils (Example 1) and **unacceptable** shortenings from hydrogenated saturated oil (Example 2).

Example 1: Acceptable Shortening

VEGETABLE SHORTENING (may contain one or more of the following partially-hydrogenated oils: soybean, corn, low erucic acid rapeseed (canola), or hydrogenated cottonseed oil.)

Example 2: Unacceptable Shortening

VEGETABLE SHORTENING (may contain one or more of the following partially-hydrogenated oils: soybean, corn, low erucic acid rapeseed (canola), **palm kernel,** or hydrogenated cottonseed oil.)

In Example 2, the addition of palm kernel oil to the list of partially-hydrogenated oil choices makes the product unacceptable.

The *Grocery Shopping Guide* classifies foods according to the type of fats they contain:

- Acceptable unsaturated, non-hydrogenated oils
- Acceptable partially-hydrogenated oils or shortenings
- Unacceptable saturated fats or shortenings

What about the total amount of fat in the diet?

The American Heart Association recommends that total fat in the diet be reduced to less than 30% of total daily calories. Fats should be distributed in the diet as follows:[33]

Saturated fat — less than 10% of total calories
Polyunsaturated fat — up to 10% of total calories
Monounsaturated fat — 10–15% of total calories

How does percent of total calories translate to grams of fat?

Most foods are labeled with the number of grams of fat per serving. Depending on your caloric intake, the following table will help you determine the total grams of fat you should be consuming per day in order to stay within the recommendations:

Calories per day	Recommended Grams of Fat			
	Total fat (30%)	Saturated fat (7–10%)	Polyun-saturated fat (up to 10%)	Monoun-saturated fat (10–15%)
1200	40	9–13	13	13–20
1500	50	11–16	16	16–25
1800	60	14–20	20	20–30
2000	66	15–22	22	22–33
2400	80	18–26	26	26–40

How do you determine percent fat calories from a product label?

Some foods are labeled with percent fat content. For example, Louis Rich Turkey Franks™ are labeled "80% fat free, 20% fat." This form of labeling often misleads the consumer to believe that this product contains only 20% of its **calories** from fat, when in reality, it actually contains 81% of its calories from fat. How can this be? It is important to know that certain foods, especially meat and poultry, are labeled with a percent of fat calculated by *weight,* not by *calories.* Although light in weight, fat is very dense in calories and supplies nine calories per gram. Therefore, a product labeled "80% fat free" means that out of a 100 grams of product, 20 grams or 180 calories (20 grams × 9 cal/gm.) are fat.

Nutrition labeling will assist you in determining the percent fat calories. For example, Louis Rich Turkey Franks™ are labeled with the following nutrition information:

Portion size	1 frank
Calories	**100**
Fat	**8 grams**
Protein	6 grams
Carbohydrate	1 gram
Sodium	480 mg.

From this information you need to note the **calories per serving** and **grams of fat per serving**. To calculate the percent calories from fat use the following formula:

$$\% \text{ calories from fat} = \frac{\text{grams fat per serving} \times 9 \text{ calories per gram}}{\text{total calories per serving}} \times 100$$

For Louis Rich Turkey Franks™, the calculation is:

$$\frac{8 \text{ grams fat per serving} \times 9 \text{ calories per gram}}{100 \text{ calories per serving}} \times 100 = .72 \times 100 = 72\%$$

This example demonstrates how a turkey frank that is labeled 80% fat free by weight actually consists of 72% fat by calories! Learning to read and decode misleading product label information is essential if you are to reduce your intake of fat and particularly saturated fat.

In the *Grocery Shopping Guide,* where deemed appropriate, foods have been classified according to their percent fat content (e.g., lunchmeat, canned spaghetti sauce and frozen dinners). It is unlikely that every single food you consume will contain less than 30% fat. **What is important is that the total day's intake provide no more than 30% fat calories.** This means that you must limit your intake of high fat foods, while consuming adequate amounts of low fat, high fiber foods.

On the following page is a sample 1500 calorie menu to help illustrate this point. As you can see, this menu contains only 18% fat which is well below the recommended 30% limit. This fat level is an average of foods consumed for the total day. Individual foods range in fat content from 0-100% fat. The key to maintaining a low fat diet is to:

- consume the majority of your calories from low fat foods such as whole grains and fruits and vegetables
- choose low fat dairy products and limited amounts of lean meats
- limit your intake of high fat foods such as vegetable oils, margarine and salad dressings.

Sample 1500 Calorie Menu

Food	Amount	Calories	Fat (gm)	% Fat*
Breakfast				
Oatmeal	1 cup	100	1.8	16
Skim milk	1 cup	86	0.4	4
Brown sugar	1 tsp.	11	0.0	0
Orange	1 med.	62	0.2	3
Lunch				
Lentil soup	1 cup	143	1.7	11
Whole grain pita bread	1/2	86	0.1	1
Tuna, water packed	2 oz.	74	0.3	3
Mayonnaise	1 tsp.	33	3.7	100
Apple	1 med.	81	0.5	6
Snack				
Oat Bran Muffin	1 muffin	127	5.1	36
Skim Milk	1 cup	86	0.4	4
Dinner				
Baked chicken (without skin)	1/2 breast	142	3.1	20
Brown rice	1/2 cup	109	0.9	7
Broccoli	1/2 cup	26	0.1	3
Whole grain roll	1	73	0.8	10
Margarine	1 tsp.	34	3.8	100
Frozen yogurt	1/2 cup	115	1.0	8
Snack				
Popcorn	3 cups	69	0.9	12
Canola oil	1 tsp.	41	4.7	100
Totals:		1498	29.5	18%

*Percent calories from fat.

Fiber — What is it, and why is everyone talking about it?

Fiber only comes from plant sources. It forms part of the outer structure of each cell. **Dietary fiber** is that portion of fruit, vegetables, whole grain cereals and other plant foods which is not broken down by the body during digestion. Diets without an adequate amount of fiber have been linked to a number of diseases including heart disease, stroke, diabetes, obesity and certain types of cancer.[1]

Preliminary studies indicate that some types of fiber may help to lower elevated blood cholesterol levels and thus may help to reduce the risk of coronary heart disease.[34]

Not all fibers are created equal. There are two types of dietary fiber:

- Water Insoluble
- Water Soluble

Water *insoluble* fibers are found in plant cell walls. They include cellulose, hemicellulose and lignin. Water *insoluble* fiber adds bulk to the diet, absorbing water and decreasing the time it takes food to move through the digestive system. This swift passage helps to prevent constipation. As a result, this type of fiber is useful in the treatment of diverticulitis, spastic colon and irritable bowel syndrome. Research also indicates a link between high fiber diets and the prevention of some types of cancer.[35] By increasing the bulk and speed of waste, *insoluble* fiber may help to dilute any carcinogens present in the lower bowel, giving them less time to do harm.

Foods that are rich sources of **water insoluble** fiber are:

Whole Grains (especially wheat)	Whole Grain Products
Brown Rice	Cereals
Vegetables (raw with peel)	Pastas
Fresh Fruit	Breads
Nuts and Seeds	Crackers

Water *soluble* fiber is the second basic type of dietary fiber. The fibers in this category include gums, psyllium and pectins, which are found in varying amounts in plants. While these fibers are useful in promoting laxation and increasing bulk, they also slow digestion and therefore delay the absorption of carbohydrates in the body. Research studies have shown beneficial effects of diets rich in water *soluble* fiber in the management of certain types of diabetes.[36,37] Water *soluble* fiber is also effective in lowering previously elevated blood cholesterol particularly if consumed along with a low cholesterol, low fat diet.[34]

Foods that are rich sources of **water soluble** fiber are:

Oats (especially oat bran)
Barley
Legumes (dry beans and peas)

Pectin-Containing Fruits
  Raw Apples
  Citrus
  Pears
  Plums

The typical American diet contains approximately 11 grams of dietary fiber per day. The National Cancer Institute recommends that Americans double their intake of fiber to 20–30 grams per day with an upper limit of 35 grams.[38]

Fiber should be consumed by eating a variety of whole grain, fresh fruits and vegetables, and dry beans and peas. Foods containing greater than 3 grams fiber per serving are marked in the *Grocery Shopping Guide* with the (★) symbol indicating that they are good sources of fiber.

Breads that list whole grains as the first ingredient and legume products are also marked with the (★) symbol, even though the fiber content is not always listed on the label.

Sodium — What is it, and how much is recommended?

Sodium is an essential mineral needed by the body to regulate blood pressure and blood volume. Sodium is also necessary for the proper functioning of nerves and muscles.

Sodium intake does not affect your blood cholesterol levels; however, excess sodium can contribute to elevated blood pressure (hypertension) in those individuals who are sodium sensitive. Hypertension is one of the major risk factors for coronary heart disease.

Most Americans consume much more sodium than they need. Several dietary surveys have reported the average daily sodium intake to range between 1800-5000 mg. per day.[39,40,41] Healthy adults under conditions of maximal adaptation and without active sweating *only* require approximately 115 mg. sodium per day. A safe **minimum** intake of 500 mg. sodium per day is set by the National Research Council (NRC).[42] This minimum requirement considers the wide variations of individuals' patterns of physical activity and climate exposure. The Food and Nutrition Board Committee recently recommended that daily intakes of sodium be limited to 2,400 mg. or less.[43] The American Heart Association recommends that sodium intake not exceed 3,000 mg. per day.[33]

What are the sources of sodium in the diet?

The major contributor of sodium to the American diet is sodium chloride (table salt). Table salt is 40% sodium and 60% chloride. A teaspoon of salt contains approximately 2,300 mg. of sodium. Sources of sodium in the typical American diet are:

- $1/3$ occurring naturally in foods
- $1/3$ added in processed foods
- $1/3$ added by cooking or at the table

How can you reduce your sodium intake?

To reduce sodium intake, reduce or eliminate the amount of salt you add to your food at the table and during cooking. Decreasing your consumption of processed foods (i.e., lunchmeats, snack foods, canned soups, and convenience foods) will also substantially reduce the sodium in your diet.

Since July 1, 1986, the United States Food and Drug Administration has required any food label that provides nutrition information to include the sodium content per serving.

Food products that provide sodium information and are high in sodium (i.e., 400 mg. or greater per serving) are identified in the *Grocery Shopping Guide* with a (▲) symbol. Products that are low in sodium (i.e., 140 mg. or less per serving) will be identified with a (▽) symbol. Unfortunately, not all food products provide sodium information. Therefore, some products may be high or low in sodium, but cannot be identified as such in the *Grocery Shopping Guide.*

It is very important to read food labels and check for salt or sodium additives as part of the ingredient list. The following is a list of high sodium food additives to watch for:

- Disodium guanylate, a flavor enhancer
- Disodium inosinate, a flavor enhancer
- Monosodium glutamate (MSG), a flavor enhancer
- Sodium benzoate, a preservative
- Sodium caseinate, a thickener and binder
- Sodium citrate, a buffer, used to control acidity in soft drinks and fruit drinks
- Sodium nitrite, a curing agent in meat, provides color, prevents botulism (a food poisoning)
- Sodium phosphate, an emulsifier, stabilizer, buffer
- Sodium propionate, a mold inhibitor
- Sodium saccharine, an artificial sweetener

The following table will help clarify sodium terminology used in nutrition labeling:

When the label says:	It means:
Sodium free	Less than 5 mg. per serving
Very low sodium	35 mg. or less per serving
Low sodium	140 mg. or less per serving
Reduced sodium	Processed to reduce the usual level of sodium by 75%
Unsalted	Processed without the normal salt used

HOW TO USE THE GROCERY SHOPPING GUIDE

The *Grocery Shopping Guide* is broken down into 12 major food groupings with 37 subclassifications (See table of contents). Individual criteria for classifying foods as **ACCEPTABLE** or **NOT RECOMMENDED** food choices have been established for each food subclassification.

Because of the unique nature of foods, certain criteria established for one type of food may not apply to another, and at first glance may seem inconsistent. For example, the butterfat content of cheese is used to determine acceptability. Low butterfat cheese is defined as containing less than 3 grams fat per ounce, medium butterfat as 4-6 grams fat per ounce, and high butterfat cheese as greater than 6 grams fat per ounce.

The criteria for classifying *cream substitutes* is different. Here low butterfat is defined as less than 2 grams fat per ounce and high butterfat as greater than 2 grams fat per ounce. The reason for this seemingly inconsistent method for classifying foods is the nature of the food and the way different food products are formulated.

Natural or processed skim milk cheeses rarely contain less than 3 grams of fat per ounce making them the lowest in fat content. Part-skim milk cheeses usually contain 4-6 grams of fat per ounce, which is considered moderate in fat and acceptable in limited quantities. All other natural or processed cheeses are high in butterfat, usually containing 7-10 grams fat per ounce and are not recommended.

When evaluating butterfat content of cream substitutes the cut-off for low fat is established at 2 grams fat per ounce. Cream substitutes containing more than 2 grams fat per ounce are considered high fat. These criteria were determined after evaluating the available cream substitutes that have been reduced in fat, without the addition of saturated tropical oils. Most of these cream substitutes contained less than 2 grams of fat per serving and therefore the criteria were so determined. If the criteria had been set consistent with those of cheese, many products with large amounts of saturated fat would have been classified as **ACCEPTABLE**.

The criteria for evaluating acceptability of the food products is therefore subjective and established by the authors to provide reasonable guidelines for selecting wise food choices. These criteria are explained at the beginning of each section.

There are literally thousands of commercially prepared foods on the grocery store shelves and hundreds of new products are introduced monthly. The *Grocery Shopping Guide* contains a large but not exhaustive sampling of foods available at the time of our survey.

The information contained in this book is correct as of the time this book was prepared for publication. However, since ingredients or processing may change from time to time, it is essential that you continue to read ingredient labels to determine how appropriate the food choices are. The criteria presented for each food classification will enable you to evaluate new and/or additional food products that were not included.

This *Guide* is not an endorsement of any single food product listed and may not be used in any form of advertising. Brand names were used solely to assist the consumer in making healthful food choices.

The following symbols will be used throughout the book to identify certain food choices.

Symbol	Key
▲	high sodium, 400 mg. or greater per serving
★	high fiber, 3 g. or greater per serving
●	contains egg yolks
▽	low sodium, 140 mg. or less per serving
✱	foot note
†	Special footnote (fat symbol)

Color Coding: Color coding has been added to this 3ᴿᴰ edition of the Grocery Shopping Guide in an attempt to make the book more user friendly. The colors green, yellow and red are used to give the criteria for evaluating foods an added dimension, further aiding the consumer in making wise food selections within each food subclassification. Criteria for evaluating foods and classifying them into **ACCEPTABLE** and **NOT RECOMMENDED** categories are explained at the beginning of each product section. Color blocks next to each criteria statement correspond to the color highlighted criteria statement at the top of the product tables.

Definitions of colors: Green: "Go"   Products coded green are the best selections under each food category. These selections are usually the lowest in saturated fat. In some sections, total fat, percent of fat calories, sodium, fiber or simple sugars may have been used in addition to saturated fat to determine the most desirable food selections.

   Green does not mean that these products can be consumed in unlimited amounts. For example, margarines coded green are the lowest in saturated fat but for the most part are 90% fat. Although these margarines are the best choices, it is recommended that they only be consumed in limited amounts.

   Yellow: "Caution"   Products coded yellow are acceptable food choices. Most products in these categories contain greater amounts of saturated fat than those coded green. In some sections, total fat, percent of fat calories, sodium, fiber or simple sugar may have been used in addition to saturated fat to determine degree of acceptability. Many of these products are recommended only in limited amounts.

   Red: "Stop"   Products coded red are those that are not recommended because they contain added sources of saturated fat or in some cases are too high in total fat or sodium.

BEVERAGES

Beverages supply the body's major source of water. Although not considered a nutrient *per se,* water is more essential to life than food itself. A person can survive for weeks without food but only a few days without water. About 50 to 65% of the adult body weight is water. To ensure adequate fluid intake, adults should consume six to eight cups of water or other beverages daily.

If chosen wisely, beverages such as unsweetened fruit or vegetable juices can contribute to good nutrition. On the other hand, beverages such as sweetened fruit drinks, soda pop and drink mixes can contribute large amounts of simple sugar to the diet.

Drinks high in simple sugar negatively affect dental health as well as create caloric excesses which often lead to obesity. Persons with diabetes, hypoglycemia or high triglycerides should limit their consumption of simple sugar.

A word of caution regarding aspartame, which is the nutritive sweetener known as Nutrasweet® or Equal®: although currently considered safe by most authorities, long-term safety has yet to be determined. Therefore, we recommend that all foods and beverages sweetened with aspartame be used in limited amounts, especially by children and pregnant women.

Some research suggests that heavy coffee consumption may be associated with increased cholesterol levels and these could predispose the drinker to atherosclerotic vascular disease.[44] Caffeine-containing beverages such as coffee, tea and cola should be limited to a maximum of 2 to 3 cups per day.

If alcoholic beverages are consumed, they should be limited to one ounce of ethanol per day. (One ounce of ethanol equals 3 ounces of 80 proof whiskey, 8 ounces of wine, or 24 ounces of beer.) Alcoholic beverage intake should be further restricted by those persons who have high triglycerides (i.e., ≥ 250 mg/dl) and those who are taking medications that may have an impact on liver function.

Beverages

ACCEPTABLE

■ **Unsweetened without added refined sugars**

Powdered drink mixes in this category contain no added refined sugars. This permits you to control both the amount and type of sweetener used. Other unsweetened frozen or ready-to-serve drinks in this category are preferred choices because they have no added refined sugars. Note that although unsweetened fruit juices contain no added refined sugars, they still contain natural simple sugars. Persons with diabetes or elevated triglyceride levels may need to restrict their intake of these products.

■ **With artificial sweetener (LIMIT USE)**

Choices in this category are artificially sweetened. Because of the lack of long term studies to determine safety, limited consumption is recommended.

■ **With added refined sugar (LIMIT USE)**

These choices may contain refined sugars such as sucrose, high fructose corn syrup, or brown sugar and are acceptable in limited amounts.

NOT RECOMMENDED

■ **With added saturated fat**

Beverages that contain added saturated fats are not recommended.

NOTE

■ Those beverages that contain added acceptable fats are identified with a (†) symbol. These fats include: soybean oil, hydrogenated and partially-hydrogenated soybean oil, cottonseed oil, partially-hydrogenated sunflower oil, corn oil, lime oil, malted milk and cocoa.

■ The sodium content of beverages varies depending on the type of beverage. Soda pop ranges from less than 5 mg. to 85 mg. sodium per 6 ounce serving. Fruit juice ranges from 0 to 15 mg. sodium per 6 ounce serving. Tomato juice and other vegetable juices range from 400-600 mg. sodium per 6 ounce serving. Milk or soy based beverages range from 85 to 180 mg. sodium per 8 ounce serving. Sodium symbols are used to indicate high (▲) or low (▽) sodium **only** when sodium content is provided on the product label. Those products that are not identified with either symbol may be either high or low sodium or contain between 141-399 mg. sodium per serving.

BRAND	ACCEPTABLE			NOT RECOMMENDED
	Unsweetened without added refined sugars	With artificial sweetener (LIMIT USE)	With added refined sugar (LIMIT USE)	With added saturated fat
CARBONATED:				
5th Avenue			▽Seltzers	
7-Up		▽Diet 7-Up ▽Diet Cherry 7-Up	7-Up Cherry 7-Up	
A&W		▽Diet cream soda ▽Diet root beer	Cream soda Root beer	
Absopure	Sparkling spring waters: ▽All flavors			

Big K		Diet soda/pop:
		  ▽All flavors
			Regular soda/pop:
			  All flavors	

Canada Dry	Club soda Seltzers: ▽All flavors	▽Diet gingerale ▽Sugar free tonic water	Gingerale Tahitian Treat Tonic water	

Canadian Spring	Premium sparkling
	  waters:
	  ▽All flavors			

Canfield's		Diet sodas:
		  ▽Cherry chocolate
		    fudge
		  ▽Chocolate fudge
		  ▽Peanut chocolate
		    fudge		

▽ Low sodium, 140 mg. or less per serving.

BRAND	ACCEPTABLE			NOT RECOMMENDED
	Unsweetened without added refined sugars	With artificial sweetener (LIMIT USE)	With added refined sugar (LIMIT USE)	With added saturated fat
Cap 10	Mineral waters: All flavors			
Chippewa	Sparkling spring water			
Coca-Cola		▽Caffeine Free Diet Coke ▽Diet Cherry Coke ▽Diet Coke	Cherry Coke Coke Coke Classic	
Country Time			▽Lemonade drink	
Crystal Geyser	Sparkling water: ▽All flavors			
Dr. Pepper		▽Diet Dr. Pepper	Dr. Pepper	
Faygo	Club soda Sparkling water: ▽All flavors	Diet soda/pop: ▽All flavors	Regular soda/pop: All flavors Tonic water	
Fresca		▽Fresca		
Hires		▽Diet root beer	Root beer	
IBC Root Beer Co.		▽Diet root beer	Root beer	
Koala Springs			Sparkling water and fruit juice: ▽All flavors	
La Croix	Sparkling pure mineral water: ▽All flavors			
Minute Maid		▽Diet orange soda	Orange soda	
Mountain Dew		▽Diet Mountain Dew	Mountain Dew	

▽ Low sodium, 140 mg. or less per serving.

Brand	Acceptable			Not Recommended
	Unsweetened without added refined sugars	**With artificial sweetener (LIMIT USE)**	**With added refined sugar (LIMIT USE)**	**With added saturated fat**
New York Seltzer		Diet New York Seltzers: ▽All flavors	New York Seltzers: ▽All flavors	
North Star	Sparkling mineral water: ▽*All flavors*			
Old San Francisco			Natural seltzers: *All flavors*	
Pepsi	▽Diet Pepsi ▽Diet Slice ▽Sugar Free Pepsi Free		Caffeine Free Pepsi Free Mandarin Orange Slice Pepsi Slice	
Perrier	Mineral waters: ▽All flavors			
R. W. Knudsen	Fruit juice spritzers: All flavors			
Robert Corr			Natural sodas: All flavors Original Ginseng Rush Sparkling Peach	
Royal Crown Cola		▽Diet Rite Cola	RC Cola	
Silver Springs	*Grapefruit seltzer water* *Natural seltzer water*			
Soho	▽*Lemon spritzer*		Cream soda Ginseng ginger ale Soho seltzers: All flavors	

▽ Low sodium, 140 mg. or less per serving.

BRAND	ACCEPTABLE			NOT RECOMMENDED
	Unsweetened without added refined sugars	With artificial sweetener (LIMIT USE)	With added refined sugar (LIMIT USE)	With added saturated fat
Sprite		▽Diet Sprite	Sprite	
Squirt		▽Diet Squirt	Squirt	
Sundance	Natural sparklers: ▽All flavors			
Sunkist		▽Diet Sunkist	Orange soda	
Swiss Creme		▽Diet soda		
Vernors		▽Diet Vernors	Vernors	
FRUIT:				
All brands	100% Unsweetened fruit juice			
After the Fall	Apple apricot Apple cherry Apple raspberry Apple strawberry Cape Cod cranberry Concord grape Georgia peach Koala punch Lemonade Maui grove Oregon berry Our original apple Pure pear Watermelon			
Awake			▽†Frozen orange beverage	

▽ Low sodium, 140 mg. or less per serving.
† Contains added acceptable fat.

BRAND	ACCEPTABLE			NOT RECOMMENDED
	Unsweetened without added refined sugars	With artificial sweetener (LIMIT USE)	With added refined sugar (LIMIT USE)	With added saturated fat
Betty Crocker			Squeezit fruit drink: ▽Cherry ▽Grape ▽Orange ▽Red punch ▽Wild berry	
Bokū			▽Fruit juice cooler	
Capri Sun			100% Natural fruit drinks and punches: All flavors	
Citrus Hill	Frozen concentrate: ▽Plus Calcium orange juice ▽Select orange juice		Frozen concentrate: Fresh recipe lemonade ▽Plus Calcium grapefruit beverage	
Cost Cutter	Apple juice Grapefruit juice Orange juice			
Country Time			▽Lemonade flavor drink	
Crystal Geyser	Juice squeeze: ▽Mountain raspberry ▽Orange and passion fruit ▽Passion fruit and mango ▽Pink lemonade ▽Wild berry			

▽ Low sodium, 140 mg. or less per serving.

BRAND	ACCEPTABLE			NOT RECOMMENDED
	Unsweetened without added refined sugars	With artificial sweetener (LIMIT USE)	With added refined sugar (LIMIT USE)	With added saturated fat

Dole	▽Pineapple orange banana juice
	▽Pineapple orange juice
	▽Pineapple-grapefruit juice
	▽Pure and Light:
	  ▽Country raspberry
	  ▽Mountain cherry
	  ▽Orchard peach
	▽Unsweetened pineapple juice			

Five Alive			Citrus beverage Frozen berry-citrus beverage Frozen citrus beverage	
General Foods			Tang: ▽Fruit beverages	
Hawaiian Punch			▽Fruit Juicy red ▽Golden passion ▽*Lite Fruit Juicy red* ▽Red grape ▽Tropical fruit ▽Wild fruit	
Health Mate	▽Natural creamed papaya juice concentrate		▽Papaya syrup juice concentrate	

▽ Low sodium, 140 mg. or less per serving.

BRAND	ACCEPTABLE			NOT RECOMMENDED
	Unsweetened without added refined sugars	With artificial sweetener (LIMIT USE)	With added refined sugar (LIMIT USE)	With added saturated fat
Hi-C			Fruit coolers: ▽All flavors Fruit drinks: ▽All flavors Fruit punch: ▽All flavors ▽Hula punch ▽Lemonade	
Indian Summer	Apple juice			
International Bazaar	*Sparkling apple cider natural apple juice* *Sparkling red grape juice natural grape juice* *Sparkling white grape juice natural grape juice*			
Kool-Aid			Koolers: ▽All flavors	
Kroger	▽Apple juice Frozen concentrate: ▽Pineapple orange juice Grape juice Grapefruit juice Orange juice ▽Pineapple juice Pink grapefruit juice Prune juice		▽Cranberry apple drink ▽Cranberry juice cocktail Frozen concentrate: ▽Cranberry juice cocktail ▽Grape juice Lemonade Limeade *Natural fruit punch* Pink lemonade	

▽ Low sodium, 140 mg. or less per serving.

BRAND	ACCEPTABLE			NOT RECOMMENDED
	Unsweetened without added refined sugars	With artificial sweetener (LIMIT USE)	With added refined sugar (LIMIT USE)	With added saturated fat
Kroger (Cont'd)			▽Raspberry cranberry juice drink	
Lakewood	Pure cranberry juice			
Libby's	Juicy juice: ▽Grape ▽Punch ▽Tropical		Apricot nectar	
Martinelli's	Apple juice ▽*Sparkling apple boysenberry* ▽Sparkling apple cranberry ▽*Sparkling apple raspberry* ▽Sparkling cider			
McCain	Junior juice: ▽Apple cherry ▽Mixed berry ▽Pure apple			
Minute Maid	100% pure juice from concentrate ▽100% pure orange juice Frozen concentrate: Apple juice Country style orange juice ▽Grapefruit ▽Orange juice		Frozen concentrate: Apple punch *Citrus punch* Country style lemonade Fruit punch Limeade ▽Pink grapefruit juice cocktail	

▽ Low sodium, 140 mg. or less per serving.

BRAND	ACCEPTABLE			NOT RECOMMENDED
	Unsweetened without added refined sugars	With artificial sweetener (LIMIT USE)	With added refined sugar (LIMIT USE)	With added saturated fat
Minute Maid (Cont'd)	Frozen concentrate (Cont'd): ▽Pulp free orange juice ▽Reduced acid orange juice		Frozen concentrate (Cont'd): Pink lemonade Regular lemonade Fruit punch	
Mott's	100% pure juice: All flavors			
Mr. Pure			Pure fruit juices and drinks: Papaya flavored drink Papaya punch	
Nice and Natural	▽Cherry delight ▽Cranberry delight Nectar and juice: ▽Passion fruit delight ▽Peach delight ▽Pina colada ▽Red raspberry delight ▽Strawberry delight			
Ocean Spray	▽100% grapefruit juice	▽Low Calorie CranApple ▽Low Calorie Cranberry juice cocktail ▽Low Calorie CranRaspberry	Juice drinks: ▽CranApple ▽Cranberry juice cocktail CranBlueberry ▽CranGrape ▽CranRaspberry ▽CranStrawberry	

▽ Low sodium, 140 mg. or less per serving.

Brand	Acceptable			Not Recommended
	Unsweetened without added refined sugars	With artificial sweetener (LIMIT USE)	With added refined sugar (LIMIT USE)	With added saturated fat
Ocean Spray (Cont'd)			Juice drinks (Cont'd): ▽Pink grapefruit juice cocktail Mauna Lai: ▽Hawaiian guava fruit drink ▽Passion fruit drink	
R.W. Knudsen	Apple cranberry Apple juice Black cherry Cherry cider Cranberry nectar Grapefruit juice Natural lemonade Payaya nectar Peach nectar Prune juice Raspberry nectar Red raspberry nectar Tropical punch			*Ambrosia* *Pineapple-coconut*
Seneca	▽Apple juice Frozen concentrated grape juice		▽Frozen cranberry juice cocktail	
Speas Farm	Apple and cherry juice Apple and raspberry juice Apple juice			
Sunny Delight			▽†Florida citrus punch	

▽ Low sodium, 140 mg. or less per serving.
† Contains added acceptable fat.

BRAND	ACCEPTABLE			NOT RECOMMENDED
	Unsweetened without added refined sugars	With artificial sweetener (LIMIT USE)	With added refined sugar (LIMIT USE)	With added saturated fat
Sunsweet	▽Prune juice ▽Prune juice (homestyle)			
Tree Sweet	Grapefruit juice Orange juice Pink grapefruit juice			
Tropicana	Frozen concentrate: Homestyle orange juice Orange juice		Twister fruit beverages	
Walkabout Springs			▽Apple and berry ▽Grapefruit ▽Lemon and lime ▽Lemon, lime and orange ▽Orange and mango	
Welch's	Sparkling red grape juice Sparkling white grape juice	No sugar added drinks: ▽Apple white grape ▽Cranberry ▽Grape juice cocktail	Frozen concentrated juice drink: ▽Cran-Raspberry juice cocktail ▽Cranberry juice cocktail Frozen concentrated sweetened: ▽100% Natural Tropicals ▽Grape juice ▽White grape juice Frozen juice cocktail: ▽Cranberry orange	

▽ Low sodium, 140 mg. or less per serving.

BRAND	ACCEPTABLE			NOT RECOMMENDED
	Unsweetened without added refined sugars	With artificial sweetener (LIMIT USE)	With added refined sugar (LIMIT USE)	With added saturated fat
Welch's (Cont'd)			Fruit juice cocktail: Apple grape Apple, grape, raspberry Apple, grape, cherry ▽Apple, orange, pineapple ▽Harvest blend ▽Grape juice Orchard: ▽Apple, orange, pineapple ▽Blended fruit juice cocktails ▽Harvest blend ▽White grape juice	
NON-CARBONATED:				
All Brands	Pure spring water			
Edensoy	Natural soy beverage: ▽†Carob ▽†Original ▽†Vanilla			
Hershey's			▽†Genuine chocolate flavored drink	

▽ Low sodium, 140 mg. or less per serving.
† Contains added acceptable fat.

BRAND	ACCEPTABLE			NOT RECOMMENDED
	Unsweetened without added refined sugars	With artificial sweetener (LIMIT USE)	With added refined sugar (LIMIT USE)	With added saturated fat
Soy Moo	▽†Non-dairy soy drink			
Sunsoy			▽†Non-dairy soy drink: *Plain*	

Westbrae Natural	West Soy:
	   ▽†Non-dairy soy drink
	 West Soy Lite:
	   Chocolate
	   Plain
	   Vanilla			

Yoo-hoo				Chocolate flavored drink
POWDERS/SYRUPS:				

All Brands	Instant coffee:
	   100% decaffeinated
	   50% decaffeinated
	   Regular
	 Instant tea:
	   Decaffeinated
	   Herbal
	   Regular			

Alba		Sugar free hot cocoa mix:
		   Chocolate and
		     marshmallow
		   Milk chocolate
				Fit-N-Frosty shake mix

Cafix	▽All natural instant beverage			

▽ Low sodium, 140 mg. or less per serving.
† Contains added acceptable fat.

BRAND	ACCEPTABLE			NOT RECOMMENDED
	Unsweetened without added refined sugars	With artificial sweetener (LIMIT USE)	With added refined sugar (LIMIT USE)	With added saturated fat
Carnation		No sugar added instant breakfast: ▽Chocolate Sugar free hot cocoa: Rich chocolate	Instant breakfast: ▽Chocolate ▽Chocolate malt ▽Strawberry ▽Vanilla	Hot cocoa mix: Chocolate fudge Chocolate with chocolate marshmallows Milk chocolate Rich chocolate Rich chocolate with marshmallows Malted milk
Classic Ovaltine			▽Traditional chocolate malt flavor	Original malt flavor
Cost Cutter				Instant cocoa mix
Country Time		Sugar free drink mix: ▽Lemonade	Drink mix: ▽Lemonade ▽Pink lemonade	
Crystal Light		Sugar free drink mixes: ▽All flavors		
Drink-Aid	Unsweetened drink mix: ▽†Fruit punch ▽Orange ▽Peach ▽Raspberry ▽Strawberry ▽†Tropical punch	Sugar free drink mix: ▽Cherry ▽Grape ▽†Orange	Sweetened drink mix: ▽Black cherry ▽Cherry ▽Cherryade ▽†Fruit punch ▽Grape ▽Grapeade ▽†Lemonade ▽Tropical punch	Sugar free drink mix: Fruit punch Lemonade Tropical punch Sweetened drink mix: *Orangeade* Unsweetened drink mix: Lemonade Pink lemonade

▽ Low sodium, 140 mg. or less per serving.
† Contains added acceptable fat.

Brand	Acceptable			Not Recommended
	Unsweetened without added refined sugars	With artificial sweetener (LIMIT USE)	With added refined sugar (LIMIT USE)	With added saturated fat
Dutch			Dutch instant cocoa mix: †Regular †With mini marshmallows	
El Molino	Cara Coa: ▽Carob powder		Cara Coa: ▽Carob drink mix	
General Foods			Tang: ▽Natural orange flavor	International coffees: Cafe amaretto Cafe Vienna *Double Dutch chocolate* *Dutch chocolate mint* Sugar free Suisse mocha Suisse mocha
Hershey			Hershey's chocolate milk mix Hershey's syrup	
Hills Brothers				Hot cocoa mix
Kaffree	Roma grain beverage			
Kool-Aid	Unsweetened soft drink mix: ▽All flavors	Sugar-free soft drink mixes: ▽All flavors	Sugar sweetened drink mix: ▽All flavors	
Kraft				Malted milk chocolate
Kroger		Light drink mix: ▽Fruit punch ▽Iced tea ▽†Lemon	*Chocolate flavored syrup* Chocolate milk mix Instant breakfast drink: All flavors	Instant coffee: Cafe amaretto Cafe Vienna Mocha supreme

▽ Low sodium, 140 mg. or less per serving.
† Contains added acceptable fat.

BRAND	ACCEPTABLE			NOT RECOMMENDED
	Unsweetened without added refined sugars	With artificial sweetener (LIMIT USE)	With added refined sugar (LIMIT USE)	With added saturated fat
Kroger (Cont'd)		Light drink mix (Cont'd): ▽Lemon-lime ▽Sugar free tea mix	Naturally sweetened tea mix ▽†Old fashioned lemonade drink mix	Instant coffee (Cont'd): Toffee Kaffee
Lipton	▽Decaffeinated iced tea mix ▽Iced tea mix	▽Sugar free iced tea mix		
Nestea	Iced tea mix	▽Sugar free iced tea mix	Lemon instant tea mix	
Nestle		Quik—sugar free: ▽†Real chocolate	Quik: Artificial strawberry flavored syrup Chocolate Chocolate flavored syrup Strawberry	Hot cocoa mix: Rich chocolate
Postum			▽Postum	
Sweet 'n Low		▽*Natural lemonade flavor drink mix Pre-sweetened instant tea: ▽†Plain ▽†With lemon		
Swiss Miss		▽†Swiss Miss sugar free hot cocoa mix	Hot cocoa mix: †Swiss Miss lite	European creme cocoa: *Amaretto creme* *Chocolate mint creme* *Chocolate mocha creme* Hot cocoa mix: Milk chocolate

▽ Low sodium, 140 mg. or less per serving.
† Contains added acceptable fat.
* Contains artificial sweetener and refined sugar.

BRAND	ACCEPTABLE			NOT RECOMMENDED
	Unsweetened without added refined sugars	With artificial sweetener (LIMIT USE)	With added refined sugar (LIMIT USE)	With added saturated fat
Swiss Miss (Cont'd)				Hot cocoa mix (Cont'd): Milk chocolate with mini-marshmallows
Wyler's	Unsweetened soft drink mix: ▽Berry burst ▽Orange ▽Red raspberry ▽Strawberry split punch ▽Tropical punch ▽Wild cherry ▽Wild grape			Unsweetened soft drink mix: Bunch o' Berries punch Lemonade
SPORT:				
Exceed			Sports nutrition supplement: †Chocolate †Vanilla	
Gatorade			▽Gatorade thirst quencher drinks	
Gear Up	▽Vitamin Gear Up			
R.W. Knudsen	Recharge thirst quenchers: ▽Lemon ▽Orange ▽Tropical			
Sports Shot			▽Sport beverage	

▽ Low sodium, 140 mg. or less per serving.
† Contains added acceptable fat.

BRAND	ACCEPTABLE			NOT RECOMMENDED
	Unsweetened without added refined sugars	With artificial sweetener (LIMIT USE)	With added refined sugar (LIMIT USE)	With added saturated fat
VEGETABLE:				
Campbell's	▲Tomato juice		▲Vegetable cocktail	
Cost Cutter	▲Tomato juice			
Heinz	Tomato juice			
Hollywood	Carrot juice			
Kroger	▲Tomato juice			
Mott's			Beefamato Clamato	
R.W. Knudsen	▲Very Veggie			
S & W	Sauerkraut juice			
V8	▽Low sodium vegetable juice ▲Spicy Hot V8 ▲Vegetable juice			

▲ High sodium, 400 mg. or greater per serving.
▽ Low sodium, 140 mg. or less per serving.

DAIRY

This section contains listings for the following food categories:
- ◇ Cheese
- ◇ Cream, Cream Substitutes, Toppings
- ◇ Milk
- ◇ Yogurt

Foods in the dairy group (especially milk, cheese and yogurt) are the body's main source of calcium, the mineral needed for the growth and repair of bones. Protein, phosphorus, B-complex vitamins (folacin, riboflavin and B12) and vitamins A and D are also supplied by dairy products. Skim milk, non-fat yogurt and skim milk cheese provide all of these nutrients with minimal amounts of butterfat.

In order to supply the body's daily requirements for these nutrients, especially calcium, it is recommended that adults consume a minimum of two servings of low fat dairy products per day. Children should consume a minimum of 3 servings per day, and teenagers and pregnant women should consume a minimum of 4 servings per day.

Cheese

ACCEPTABLE

■ **Low butterfat cheese, 3 grams or less fat per ounce or ¼ cup**
Choices from this category are the most desirable because they contain the least amount of saturated fat.

▨ **Medium butterfat cheese, 4-6 grams of fat per ounce or ¼ cup (LIMIT USE)**
Although these products contain reduced amounts of saturated fat, they still contain a significant amount of fat and should be used sparingly. Cheese from this category contain as much saturated fat as equal portions of red meat.

▨ **Cheese substitute, cheese made with partially hydrogenated oil (LIMIT USE)**
Products in this category are usually labeled "imitation cheese, no cholesterol." The animal fat (i.e., butterfat) has been taken out and replaced with partially hydrogenated vegetable oil (usually soybean oil). Note these products are **not** low in fat, and some are fairly high in sodium. Limited intake is recommended.

NOT RECOMMENDED

■ **High butterfat cheese, greater than 6 grams of fat per ounce or ¼ cup**
These cheeses usually contain 7-10 grams of fat (mostly saturated) per ounce.

NOTE

- The sodium content of natural cheese is significantly lower than that of processed cheese. Natural cheese ranges from 150-200 mg. sodium per 1 ounce serving. Processed cheese ranges from 300-400 mg. sodium per 1 ounce serving. Sodium symbols are used to indicate high (▲) or low (▽) sodium **only** when sodium content is provided on the product label. Those products that are not identified with either symbol may be either high or low sodium or contain between 141-399 mg. sodium per serving.

BRAND	ACCEPTABLE			NOT RECOMMENDED
	Low butterfat cheese, 3 grams or less fat per oz. or ¼ cup	†Medium butterfat cheese, 4-6 grams of fat per oz. or ¼ cup (LIMIT USE)	Cheese substitute, cheese made with partially hydrogenated oil (LIMIT USE)	High butterfat cheese, greater than 6 grams of fat per oz. or ¼ cup

All brands	Cottage cheese:
	1% low fat
	2% low fat
	Dry curd
				Blue
				Brick
				Brie
				Camembert
				Caraway
				*Cheddar
				Cheshire
				*Colby
				Cottage cheese:
				   Creamed 4% fat
				*Cream cheese
				Edam
				*Farmer's cheese
				*Feta
				Fontina
				Frankenmuth
				Gjetost
				Gouda
				Gruyere
				Limburger
				Monterey Jack
				Mozzarella:
				   *Whole milk
				Muenster

* Certain specially processed lowfat varieties are available. See brand name listings.
**Limited amounts of grated cheese are allowed.
† Medium butterfat cheeses have been reduced in fat but are still high in saturated fat, use sparingly.

BRAND	ACCEPTABLE			NOT RECOMMENDED
	Low butterfat cheese, 3 grams or less fat per oz. or ¼ cup	†Medium butterfat cheese, 4-6 grams of fat per oz. or ¼ cup (LIMIT USE)	Cheese substitute, cheese made with partially hydrogenated oil (LIMIT USE)	High butterfat cheese, greater than 6 grams of fat per oz. or ¼ cup
All brands (Cont'd)	Grated parmesan (limit 2 Tbsp.) Grated romano (limit 2 Tbsp.)	Ricotta: Part-skim		Neufchatel **Parmesan Pinconning Port du salut Processed cheese spread Provolone Ricotta: *Whole milk **Romano Roquefort *Swiss
Alouette				Soft spreadable cheese garlic and spices
Alpine Lace	Free N' Lean: Fat free, low cholesterol	American flavor, pasteurized process cheese product ▽Ched-R-Lo, Part-skim milk cheese ▽Colbi-Lo, Part-skim semisoft cheese ▽Monti-Jack-Lo, Part-skim milk cheese ▽Mozzarella Cheese, Low Moisture part-skim		Muenster, Low sodium

▽ Low sodium, 140 mg. or less per serving.
 * Certain specially processed lowfat varieties are available. See brand name listings.
**Limited amounts of grated cheese are allowed.
 † Medium butterfat cheeses have been reduced in fat but are still high in saturated fat, use sparingly.

BRAND	ACCEPTABLE			NOT RECOMMENDED
	Low butterfat cheese, 3 grams or less fat per oz. or ¼ cup	†Medium butterfat cheese, 4-6 grams of fat per oz. or ¼ cup (LIMIT USE)	Cheese substitute, cheese made with partially hydrogenated oil (LIMIT USE)	High butterfat cheese, greater than 6 grams of fat per oz. or ¼ cup
Alpine Lace (Cont'd)		▽Provo-Lo, Litely smoked part-skim milk cheese ▽Swiss-Lo, Part-skim milk cheese		
Alta-Dena				Kefir cheese Natural Monterey Jack cheese
Andrulis				Farmer's cheese Feta cheese
Andrys				Farmer's cheese
Baker		String cheese		

Borden	Lite line:
	    American
	    Colby
	    Sharp cheddar
	    Swiss
		Light American flavor	Lite line:
			    ▲Low cholesterol
				All other natural, processed or imitation cheese food or spread

Casino		Natural low moisture part-skim mozzarella		Muenster cheese
Cost Cutter				‡Process cheese food ‡Shredded pizza topping
County Line		100% natural, part-skim mozzarella string cheese American Pasteurized Process Cheese Food		Medium sharp cheddar Mild Colby Monterey Jack Sharp cheddar

▲ High sodium, 400 mg. or greater per serving.
‡ Contains added palm oil.
† Medium butterfat cheeses have been reduced in fat but are still high in saturated fat, use sparingly.

BRAND	ACCEPTABLE			NOT RECOMMENDED
	Low butterfat cheese, 3 grams or less fat per oz. or ¼ cup	†Medium butterfat cheese, 4-6 grams of fat per oz. or ¼ cup (LIMIT USE)	Cheese substitute, cheese made with partially hydrogenated oil (LIMIT USE)	High butterfat cheese, greater than 6 grams of fat per oz. or ¼ cup
County Line (Cont'd)		Part-skim mozzarella (Shredded)		
Cracker Barrel				Cold pack cheese food, sharp Extra Sharp cheddar Medium cheddar Sharp cheddar
Delicia			American and caraway cheese American and hot pepper cheese American processed cheese substitute ▲Hickory smoked American cheese	
Dorman's		Light: Lo-Chol ▽Reduced fat cheddar cheese	▽Muenster cheese alternative	Light: *Chedda-Delight* *Slim Jack* Swiss, low sodium
Fischer			Ched-O-Mate: Imitation cheddar cheese	

▲ High sodium, 400 mg. or greater per serving.
▽ Low sodium, 140 mg. or less per serving.
† Medium butterfat cheeses have been reduced in fat but are still high in saturated fat, use sparingly.

BRAND	ACCEPTABLE			NOT RECOMMENDED
	Low butterfat cheese, 3 grams or less fat per oz. or ¼ cup	†Medium butterfat cheese, 4-6 grams of fat per oz. or ¼ cup (LIMIT USE)	Cheese substitute, cheese made with partially hydrogenated oil (LIMIT USE)	High butterfat cheese, greater than 6 grams of fat per oz. or ¼ cup
Fischer (Cont'd)			Pizza Mate: Imitation mozzarella cheese ▲Sandwich Mate	
Fleur de Lait		▽Ultra Light spreadable cheese with berries		
Formagg			▽No cholesterol, no lactose cheese substitute	
Frigo	Grated parmesan (limit 2 Tbsp.) Grated Romano cheese (limit 2 Tbsp.) ▽Part-skim ricotta	Part-skim mozzarella		Feta (shredded) Parmesan Ricotta: Whole milk Romano Shredded provolone
Gamay	Cheese Smart Pasteurized process cheese: ▲Individual sliced cheese Cheese Smart skim milk cheese product: Cheddar flavor (block/shredded) ▲Mozzarella flavor (shredded)			

▲ High sodium, 400 mg. or greater per serving.
▽ Low sodium, 140 mg. or less per serving.
† Medium butterfat cheeses have been reduced in fat but are still high in saturated fat, use sparingly.

BRAND	ACCEPTABLE			NOT RECOMMENDED
	Low butterfat cheese, 3 grams or less fat per oz. or ¼ cup	†Medium butterfat cheese, 4-6 grams of fat per oz. or ¼ cup (LIMIT USE)	Cheese substitute, cheese made with partially hydrogenated oil (LIMIT USE)	High butterfat cheese, greater than 6 grams of fat per oz. or ¼ cup
Jarlsburg				Semi-soft part-skim cheese
Kau Kauna				Cold pack cheese food: Extra sharp cheddar
Kraft		Light n' Lively: ▲American Light Naturals: Colby Mild cheddar Monterey Jack *Swiss* Low moisture, part-skim mozzarella Shredded, low moisture mozzarella and provolone String cheese		All other natural, processed or imitation cheese food or spread Pimento single slices Single slices Swiss
Kroger	Cottage cheese: Lowfat, 2% Nonfat Lite Classics: ▽Reduced calorie mozzarella cheese (shredded) ▽Ricotta	▲American Light Lite Classics: ▽Reduced calorie mild cheddar cheese (shredded) Low moisture part-skim mozzarella Nice n' Cheesy		All other natural, processed or imitation cheese food or spread Cottage cheese: Large curd, 4% Small curd, 4% Squeeze cheese: All flavors

▲ High sodium, 400 mg. or greater per serving.
▽ Low sodium, 140 mg. or less per serving.
† Medium butterfat cheeses have been reduced in fat but are still high in saturated fat, use sparingly.

Brand	Acceptable			Not Recommended
	Low butterfat cheese, 3 grams or less fat per oz. or ¼ cup	†Medium butterfat cheese, 4-6 grams of fat per oz. or ¼ cup (LIMIT USE)	Cheese substitute, cheese made with partially hydrogenated oil (LIMIT USE)	High butterfat cheese, greater than 6 grams of fat per oz. or ¼ cup
Land O Lakes		American singles		
Laughing Cow	Reduced calorie wedge	Cheddar cheese wedges *Reduced calorie mini bonbel*		Baby Bel Mini bonbel Mini gouda
Lorraine Lites		▽Mozzarella, Low Moisture, Part-Skim ▽Reduced Fat Cheddar ▽Reduced Fat Colby ▽Reduced Fat Monterey Jack ▽Reduced Fat Muenster ▽Reduced Fat Provolone ▽Reduced Fat Swiss		
Marlas				Very low sodium, low cholesterol natural semi-hard part-skim milk cheese
May Bud	*Part-skim milk parmesan cheese (limit 2 Tbsp. grated)*	*Diet snack, cheese food product:* *Cheddar* *Sharp cheddar* Farmer's cheese, semi-soft, skim		All other natural, processed or imitation cheese food or spread Caraway gouda Edam French onion hickory gouda

▽ Low sodium, 140 mg. or less per serving.
† Medium butterfat cheeses have been reduced in fat but are still high in saturated fat, use sparingly.

BRAND	ACCEPTABLE			NOT RECOMMENDED
	Low butterfat cheese, 3 grams or less fat per oz. or ¼ cup	†Medium butterfat cheese, 4-6 grams of fat per oz. or ¼ cup (LIMIT USE)	Cheese substitute, cheese made with partially hydrogenated oil (LIMIT USE)	High butterfat cheese, greater than 6 grams of fat per oz. or ¼ cup
May Bud (Cont'd)				Gouda Hickory smoked edam Monterey Jack cheese
Merkts				All cheese spreads
Miceli's	▽Part-skim ricotta	Low moisture part-skim mozzarella		
Nu Tofu			*Natural cheese*	
NUCOA			Heart Beat cholesterol free cheese	

Philadelphia		§Light cream cheese (soft/tub)		Cream cheese:
				    Chives and onion
				    Cream cheese and pineapple
				    Regular:
				        (soft/tub)
				Light neufchatel cheese

Sargento	▽Lite ricotta
	▽Moo Town Snacker:
	    Lite String cheese
		Moo Town Snacker:
		    String cheese
		Shredded part-skim mozzarella
				Limburger
				Moo Town Snacker:
				    Mild cheddar

Schuler's				Cheese spread

▽ Low sodium, 140 mg. or less per serving.
§ Cream cheese contains less protein and calcium than other cheeses.
† Medium butterfat cheeses have been reduced in fat but are still high in saturated fat, use sparingly.

BRAND	ACCEPTABLE			NOT RECOMMENDED
	Low butterfat cheese, 3 grams or less fat per oz. or ¼ cup	†Medium butterfat cheese, 4-6 grams of fat per oz. or ¼ cup (LIMIT USE)	Cheese substitute, cheese made with partially hydrogenated oil (LIMIT USE)	High butterfat cheese, greater than 6 grams of fat per oz. or ¼ cup
Springsdale Farms		Lite Classic reduced calorie pasteurized processed American cheese		
Stella		*Low moisture, part-skim mozzarella*		
Swiss Knight				Fondue cheese
Swiss Lorraine				Swiss cheese
Tiger				Gruyere wedges
Tofu Rella			Jalapeno Jack Mozzarella Natural Monterey Jack style	
Treasure Cave				Blue cheese
Velveeta		▲Processed cheese spreads		
Weight Watchers	Pasteurized process cheese product: ▲American Sharp cheddar flavor ▽§*Reduced calorie cream cheese spread*	*Cold pack cheese food* ▽Natural colby flavor cheese ▽Natural mozzarella soft part-skim cheese Natural part-skim cheese		

▲ High sodium, 400 mg. or greater per serving.
▽ Low sodium, 140 mg. or less per serving.
§ Cream cheese contains less protein and calcium than other cheeses.
† Medium butterfat cheeses have been reduced in fat but are still high in saturated fat, use sparingly.

Cream, Cream Substitutes, Toppings

ACCEPTABLE

■ **No fat or contain acceptable oil, may be partially hydrogenated (LIMIT USE)**
These products are better choices because they do not contain animal fat (i.e., butterfat). Some products are, however, high in fat and should be used in limited amounts. These products are not appropriate as milk substitutes.

■ **Low butterfat, 2 grams or less fat per ounce (LIMIT USE)**
These products contain butterfat but in reduced amounts. They may be acceptable in limited amounts. These products are not appropriate as milk substitutes.

NOT RECOMMENDED

■ **High butterfat, greater than 2 grams fat per ounce or with added tropical oils**
Food products with greater than 2 grams butterfat per ounce are considered high butterfat and are not recommended. Products containing coconut, palm, or palm kernel oil are also not recommended.

NOTE

■ Products in this category contain between 0 to 15 mg. sodium per 1 ounce serving. Sodium symbols are used to indicate high (▲) or low (▽) sodium **only** when sodium content is provided on the product label. Those products that are not identified with either symbol may be either high or low sodium or contain between 141-399 mg. sodium per serving.

BRAND	ACCEPTABLE		NOT RECOMMENDED
	No fat or contain acceptable oil, may be partially hydrogenated (LIMIT USE)	Low butterfat, 2 grams or less fat per oz. (LIMIT USE)	High butterfat, greater than 2 grams fat per oz. or with added tropical oils
FRESH:			
All brands			Cream Half and half Sour cream Whipping cream
Borden			100% real half and half
Breakstones		▽Light choice sour cream	Sour cream
C.F. Burger			Half-and-half creamer

Carnation	Coffee-Mate:
	  ▽Liquid non-dairy creamer
	  ▽Light non-dairy liquid
	    creamer		

Encore			Sour cream substitute
Farm Rich	Light non-dairy breakfast creamer Non-dairy breakfast creamer		
Kroger		▽Lite 'n Sour ▽Real whipped light cream	
Land O Lakes		▽Light sour cream	
Light n' Lively Free	Nonfat sour cream alternative		
Melody Farms			Half and half
Mocha mix	▽Non-dairy creamer		
Presto Whip			*Non-dairy whipped topping*

▽ Low sodium, 140 mg. or less per serving.

Brand	Acceptable		Not Recommended
	No fat or contain acceptable oil, may be partially hydrogenated (LIMIT USE)	**Low butterfat, 2 grams or less fat per oz. (LIMIT USE)**	**High butterfat, greater than 2 grams fat per oz. or with added tropical oils**
Reddi Whip			Deluxe real heavy whipped cream Real whipped light cream
Rich's			Rich Whip non-dairy whipped topping
Sealtest			½ and ½ singles
Weight Watchers		▽Sour cream style blend	
FROZEN:			
Cool Whip			Cool Whip: 　Extra creamy whipped topping 　Regular whipped topping Cool Whip Lite: 　Whipped topping
Kroger			Extra creamy whipped topping Non-dairy creamer Non-dairy whipped topping
Nature's Best			Non-dairy whipped topping
Pet Inc.			LaCreme: 　Whipped topping
Rich's	▽Coffee Rich		

▽ Low sodium, 140 mg. or less per serving.

BRAND	ACCEPTABLE		NOT RECOMMENDED
	No fat or contain acceptable oil, may be partially hydrogenated (LIMIT USE)	Low butterfat, 2 grams or less fat per oz. (LIMIT USE)	High butterfat, greater than 2 grams fat per oz. or with added tropical oils
POWDERS:			
Borden	Cremora Lite: ▽Non-dairy creamer		Cremora non-dairy creamer
Carnation	Coffee-Mate: ▽Lite Non-dairy creamer		Coffee-Mate: Regular
Cost Cutter	▽Non-dairy creamer		
D-Zerta			Reduced calorie whipped topping mix
Dream Whip			Whipped topping mix
Estee			Whipped topping mix
Kroger			Non-dairy creamer Whipped topping mix
Weight Watchers	▽*Dairy creamer		

▽ Low sodium, 140 mg. or less per serving.
* Contains no fat.

Milk

■ **Nonfat, less than 1 gram of fat per serving**
Skim milk products having only trace amounts of saturated fat are the preferred choices.

■ **Low fat, 2.5 grams of fat or less per serving**
Listed in this category are 1/2% and 1% low fat milk products. These products contain 1-3 grams of fat per 8 ounces.

NOT RECOMMENDED

■ **High-fat, greater than 2.5 grams fat per serving**
These milks contain 5-8 grams of fat per 8 ounce serving and include all whole milk and 2% milk products.

NOTE

■ Most fresh milk contains between 120-130 mg. sodium per 8 ounce serving with the exception of buttermilk which contains approximately 260 mg. per 8 ounce serving. Sodium symbols are used to indicate high (▲) or low (▽) sodium **only** when sodium content is provided on the product label. Those products that are not identified with either symbol may be either high or low sodium or contain between 141-399 mg. sodium per serving.

BRAND	ACCEPTABLE		NOT RECOMMENDED
	Nonfat, less than 1 gran of fat per serving	Low fat, 2.5 grams of fat or less per serving	High fat, greater than 2.5 grams fat per serving
All brands	Evaporated skim milk Nonfat dry milk Skim milk	1% milk 1/2% milk	2% milk Whole milk
Alba	Instant nonfat dry milk, high calcium		Fit-N-Frosty Shake powder
Alta-Dena			*Strawberry cultured milk*
Borden			Eagle brand sweetened condensed milk
C. F. Burger	Lactaid, Nonfat		Old fashioned egg nog
Calci-Milk		▽Calci-milk with lactaid	
Carnation	Nonfat dry milk powder		Evaporated milk Sweetened condensed milk
Cost Cutter			Evaporated milk
Hershey			Chocolate milk
Kroger	▽Nonfat dry milk	Cultured lowfat buttermilk, 1%	2% milk Chocolate milk, 2% Evaporated milk
Longlife		▽Lactaid brand 1% milk	
Nestle			Quik chocolate milk Quik strawberry milk
Old Fashioned			Instant egg nog mix
Periwinkle			100% natural Swiss goat's milk

▽ Low sodium, 140 mg. or less per serving.

BRAND	ACCEPTABLE		NOT RECOMMENDED
	Nonfat, less than 1 gram of fat per serving	Low fat, 2.5 grams of fat or less per serving	High fat, greater than 2.5 grams fat per serving
Pet Inc.	Light, evaporated, low cholesterol, low fat skimmed milk		Evaporated milk
Saco	Cultured buttermilk blend dry buttermilk powder		
Sealtest		▽Sweet Acidophilus lowfat milk	
Vitamite			Lactose free non-dairy beverage

▽ Low sodium, 140 mg. or less per serving.

Yogurt

ACCEPTABLE

■ **1% fat or less**
These products are the best choices and contain 2 grams of fat or less per 8 ounce serving.

□ **1.5% fat**
These are also acceptable choices but are slightly higher in fat, usually containing 3 grams of fat per 8 ounce serving.

NOT RECOMMENDED

■ **2% fat or greater and/or with added saturated fat**
Those products containing 2% fat or greater are considered high in fat and are not recommended.

NOTE

■ Some yogurts are high in sugar content. Those individuals monitoring their sugar or caloric intake may want to assess simple sugar as well as fat content of yogurt. Many low calorie yogurts contain artificial sweeteners such as Nutrasweet or saccharine, see page 31 for recommendations regarding use of artificial sweeteners.

■ The sodium content of yogurt ranges between 95-160 mg. per 8 ounce serving. Sodium symbols are used to indicate high (▲) or low (▽) sodium **only** when sodium content is provided on the product label. Those products that are not identified with either symbol may be either high or low sodium or contain between 141-399 mg. sodium per serving.

BRAND	ACCEPTABLE		NOT RECOMMENDED
	1% fat or less	1.5% fat	2% fat or greater and/or with added saturated fat
All brands	1% fat or less	1.5% fat	2% fat or greater
Breyers	Lowfat yogurt: ▽Black cherry ▽Blueberry ▽Mixed berry ▽Raspberry ▽Strawberry/banana		Yogurt: All flavors (2% fat or greater)
Colombo	Non-fat Lite: ▽All flavors		Regular yogurt
Dannon	Fruit on the bottom yogurt (1% fat): All flavors Light nonfat yogurt: ▽All flavors Light nonfat yogurt with aspartame sweetener: ▽All flavors ▽Nonfat plain yogurt	▽Fresh flavors Lowfat yogurt: Plain Lowfat yogurt (1.5%): ▽All flavors	Blended with fruit yogurt (2% fat): All flavors Lowfat yogurt: Pina colada
Espirit	*Custard style breakfast yogurt* Lowfat yogurt: *All flavors* Nonfat yogurt: All flavors		*Extra smooth*
Kissle			Creamy blend yogurt: All flavors

▽ Low sodium, 140 mg. or less per serving.

Brand	Acceptable		Not Recommended
	1% fat or less	1.5% fat	2% fat or greater and/or with added saturated fat

Kroger	Kroger Lite reduced calorie non-fat yogurt:
	    All flavors (1% fat or less)
	Lowfat yogurt:
	    ▽Fruit flavors
		Lowfat yogurt:
		    Plain
		    Vanilla
			Lowfat yogurt:
			    Pina colada

LaYogurt			Yogurt: All flavors

Light n' Lively	Lowfat yogurt:
	    ▽All flavors (1% fat or less)
	Nonfat yogurt with aspartame:
	    ▽All flavors		

Mountain High	Honey light natural yoghurt: Strawberry		Plain and flavored natural yoghurt
Stir Fruity			*All flavors*
Tuscan Farms	Lowfat yogurt drink: ▽*All flavors*		
Weight Watchers	Nonfat yogurt: ▽*All flavors* ▽Ultimate nonfat yogurt		

Yoplait	Fat free "150":
	    ▽*All flavors*
	Light nonfat yogurt:
	    ▽All flavors
		Original lowfat yogurt:
		    ▽Fruit Flavors
			Breakfast style
			Custard style yogurt:
			    All flavors
			Original pina colada

Yubi	Lowfat yogurt:
	    ▽Fruit flavors
	    Plain
	    ▽Vanilla		

▽ Low sodium, 140 mg. or less per serving.

EGGS

Egg whites are an excellent source of protein and contain no cholesterol. The yolk is particularly rich in phosphorous, sulfur, iron and vitamin A, but unfortunately provides the single most concentrated source of cholesterol in the American diet (213 mg. per yolk). The American Heart Association recommends that you consume no more than four egg yolks per week, including those used in cooking.

Here are some tips for decreasing your egg yolk consumption:

- Modify recipes calling for whole eggs by substituting two egg whites in place of one whole egg.

- Prepare a three egg omelette by using two egg whites and one whole egg.

- Prepare your own egg substitute by combining one egg white with 2¼ tsp. nonfat dry milk powder and 1 tsp. canola oil. Combine ingredients in a blender. (Yield is equivalent to one egg.)

- Experiment using steamed tofu (soybean curd), which has a consistency very much like egg white. It can be used to make an "eggless" egg salad.

- Use commercially prepared egg substitutes that are cholesterol free (see p. 75).

Egg Substitutes

ACCEPTABLE

■ **Contains no cholesterol**
Acceptable choices are those egg substitutes that contain no cholesterol.

NOT RECOMMENDED

■ **Contains cholesterol or added saturated fat**
Egg substitutes containing cholesterol are not recommended.

NOTE

■ Sodium content of a fresh whole egg is 69 mg. with the egg white containing 50 mg. Egg substitutes contain between 80-180 mg. sodium per 4 ounce serving. Sodium symbols are used to indicate high (▲) or low (▽) sodium **only** when sodium content is provided on the product label. Those products that are not identified with either symbol may be either high or low sodium or contain between 141-399 mg. sodium per serving.

BRAND	ACCEPTABLE	NOT RECOMMENDED
	Contains No Cholesterol	Contains Cholesterol or added Saturated fat
Fleischmann's	▽Egg Beaters Egg Beaters vegetable omelette	Egg Beaters with Cheez
Healthy Choice	Cholesterol free egg product	
Kroger	▽Kroger egg substitute	
Land O Lakes		*Country Morning* *Scrambled*
Morning Star Farms	▽Scramblers	
Second Nature	▽*Imitation eggs* ▽No cholesterol egg product	

▽ Low sodium, 140 mg. or less per serving.

ETHNIC FOODS

This section contains listings for the following food categories:

◇ Italian
◇ Kosher
◇ Mexican
◇ Oriental

Ethnic foods offer variety in the diet and in many cases can be wholesome and nutritious. Processed ethnic foods, however, often contain excessive amounts of fat and sodium. When possible it is always better to prepare these foods from scratch so that you can control the type and amount of ingredients used. The following selections of foods have been evaluated by type and amount of fat contained. Foods known to be high in sodium (i.e., greater than 400 mg. per serving) are identified by a (▲) symbol. Since sodium information is not available for all products, some foods high in sodium may not be identified.

Italian

ACCEPTABLE

■ **With added acceptable ingredients* and 30% or less calories from fat**
Choices from this category are the most desirable because they contain the least amount of fat.

■ **With added acceptable ingredients*, greater than 30% fat (but less than 6 grams fat per serving) or fat per serving is unknown (LIMIT USE)**
Products in this category contain acceptable ingredients but are either higher in fat or are not labeled with nutrition information in order to determine the quantity or percent of fat. To help distinguish the products with questionable fat content, a (†) symbol will identify those with missing nutrition labeling. Since these products may be high in fat (i.e. 6 or more grams fat per serving) limited intake is recommended.

NOT RECOMMENDED

■ **6 or more grams fat per serving or contains added saturated fats**
Products containing 6 or more grams of fat per serving or containing added saturated fat are not recommended.

NOTE

■ Most foods in this section are high in sodium and can range from 300-900 mg. per serving. Sodium symbols are used to indicate high (▲) or low (▽) sodium **only** when sodium content is provided on the product label. Those products that are not identified with either symbol may be either high or low sodium or contain between 141-399 mg. sodium per serving.

*Acceptable ingredients include all unsaturated oils or added meat or cheese.

BRAND	ACCEPTABLE		NOT RECOMMENDED
	With added acceptable ingredients and 30% or less calories from fat	With added acceptable ingredients greater than 30% fat (but less than 6 g fat per serving) or fat/serving is unknown (LIMIT USE)	6 or more grams fat per serving or contains added saturated fats
Appian Way			Pizza dinner, regular
Buitoni		Spaghetti sauce: †*Marinara* †Meatless †Mushroom	
Chef Boyardee	▲Complete spaghetti dinner ▲Dinosaurs, cheese flavor Microwave meals: 　▲Dinosaurs in spaghetti sauce — cheese flavor 　▲Tic Tac Toe with spaghetti sauce — cheese flavor Mini ravioli ▲Tic Tac Toe in spaghetti sauce with cheese flavor	Microwave meals: †Cheese ravioli in tomato and meat sauce †Dinosaurs with mini meatballs in tomato sauce †Elbows and beef in sauce †Lasagna in garden vegetable sauce †Pasta shells in tomato and meat sauce †Pasta shells in tomato sauce with mushrooms †Rigatoni — pasta in tomato and meat sauce Pizza mix: †Cheese Sharks: †Pasta shapes and mini meatballs in tomato sauce	Beef ravioli Beefaroni Complete lasagna dinner Dinosaurs with meatballs in tomato sauce Lasagna pasta and beef in sauce Microwave meals: 　Beef ravioli in tomato and meat sauce 　Beefaroni 　Lasagna in beef sauce 　Spaghetti and meatballs in tomato sauce 　Tic Tac Toe with mini meatballs in tomato sauce Mini canneloni Pac Man: 　In golden chicken flavored sauce

▲ High sodium, 400 mg. or greater per serving.
† Fat per serving unknown, limit use.

BRAND	ACCEPTABLE		NOT RECOMMENDED
	With added acceptable ingredients and 30% or less calories from fat	With added acceptable ingredients greater than 30% fat (but less than 6 g fat per serving) or fat/serving is unknown (LIMIT USE)	6 or more grams fat per serving or contains added saturated fats
Chef Boyardee (Cont'd)		Sharks (Cont'd): †Pasta shapes in spaghetti sauce — cheese flavor	Spaghetti with meatballs Tic Tac Toe with meatballs in tomato sauce
Classico		†Beef and pork spaghetti sauce †Olive and mushroom spaghetti sauce Pasta sauce: †Red pepper †Shrimp and crab †Tomato and basil spaghetti sauce	
Contadina		Pizza sauce: †Original flavor Pizza squeeze: †Pizza sauce	
Cost Cutter		Spaghetti sauce: †Flavored with meat †Regular †With mushrooms	

† Fat per serving unknown, limit use.

BRAND	ACCEPTABLE		NOT RECOMMENDED
	With added acceptable ingredients and 30% or less calories from fat	**With added acceptable ingredients greater than 30% fat (but less than 6 g fat per serving) or fat/serving is unknown (LIMIT USE)**	**6 or more grams fat per serving or contains added saturated fats**
Domino's Pizza	Spaghetti sauce: ▲Meat flavor ▲Original ▲With mushrooms		
Enrico's	Spaghetti sauce: All natural No salt added With mushrooms	Pizza sauce: †All natural	
Estee		*Beef ravioli*	*Spaghetti and meatballs*
Franco American	▲Macaroni and cheese ▲Spaghetti in tomato sauce ▲Spaghetti O's in tomato and cheese sauce ▲Sport O's in tomato and cheese sauce ▲Teddy O's in tomato and cheese sauce	†Beefy mac	Beef Ravioli O's in meat sauce Spaghetti O's with meatballs in tomato sauce Spaghetti O's with sliced franks in tomato sauce Spaghetti with meatballs in tomato sauce Sport O's with meatballs in tomato sauce Teddy O's with meatballs in tomato sauce

▲ High sodium, 400 mg. or greater per serving.
† Fat per serving unknown, limit use.

BRAND	ACCEPTABLE		NOT RECOMMENDED
	With added acceptable ingredients and 30% or less calories from fat	With added acceptable ingredients greater than 30% fat (but less than 6 g fat per serving) or fat/serving is unknown (LIMIT USE)	6 or more grams fat per serving or contains added saturated fats
Hunt's	Spaghetti sauce: ▲Chunky style ▲Homestyle ▲Meat ▲Mushroom ▲Traditional		
Jiffy			Pizza crust mix
Kraft	*Spaghetti dinner* ▲Tangy Italian style dinner		
Kroger	▲Beef ravioli Chunky style spaghetti sauce: ▲Extra tomato, garlic and onions ▲Green peppers and mushrooms ▲Mushrooms and onions Homestyle 100% natural sauce: ▲Meat ▲Mushroom ▲Traditional Spaghetti sauce: ▲Meat	Pizza sauce: †Pepperoni flavored †Sausage flavored †Traditional †With mushrooms Spaghetti sauce: †Mushroom	Spaghetti sauce: Traditional

▲ High sodium, 400 mg. or greater per serving.
† Fat per serving unknown, limit use.

BRAND	ACCEPTABLE		NOT RECOMMENDED
	With added acceptable ingredients and 30% or less calories from fat	With added acceptable ingredients greater than 30% fat (but less than 6 g fat per serving) or fat/serving is unknown (LIMIT USE)	6 or more grams fat per serving or contains added saturated fats
Lunch Bucket	Beef ravioli in meat sauce ▲Lasagna with meat and sauce		
Martha White			Pizza crust mix
Nature's Best		Spaghetti sauce: †*Meat flavor* †*Meatless*	
Newman's Own		Spaghetti sauce: †Traditional †With mushrooms	
Prego		Extra chunky spaghetti sauce: ▲Mushroom and onion ▲Mushroom and tomato Spaghetti sauce: ▲Fresh mushrooms	Extra chunky spaghetti sauce: Mushroom and green pepper Tomato, onion and garlic Spaghetti sauce: No salt added Plain With meat
Pritikin	Spaghetti sauce: ▽Regular ▽With mushrooms		

▲ High sodium, 400 mg. or greater per serving.
▽ Low sodium, 140 mg. or less per serving.
† Fat per serving unknown, limit use.

BRAND	ACCEPTABLE		NOT RECOMMENDED
	With added acceptable ingredients and 30% or less calories from fat	With added acceptable ingredients greater than 30% fat (but less than 6 g fat per serving) or fat/serving is unknown (LIMIT USE)	6 or more grams fat per serving or contains added saturated fats

Progresso		▲Marinara sauce
		Spaghetti sauce:
		  †Meat flavor
		  †Red clam
		  †White clam	

Ragu	100% Natural old world style:
	  ▲Meat flavored
	Chunky garden style spaghetti sauce:
	  ▲Extra tomatoes, garlic and onions
	  ▲Mushroom and green pepper
	  ▲Mushroom and onions
	Homestyle 100% natural spaghetti sauce:
	  Flavored with meat
	  Mushroom
	  Plain
	Original style 100% natural spaghetti sauce:
	  ▲With meat
	Quick pizza crust
		100% Natural old world style:
		  ▲Mushroom
		  ▲Plain
		100% natural pizza sauce
		Fresh Italian 100% natural pasta sauce:
		  ▲Parmesan
		  ▲Sliced mushroom
		  ▲Tomato and herbs
		  ▲Zesty tomato
		Original style 100% natural spaghetti sauce:
		  ▲Original
		Pizza Quick sauce:
		  Flavored with cheese
		  Traditional
			Pizza Quick sauce:
			  Flavored with pepperoni

▲ High sodium, 400 mg. or greater per serving.
† Fat per serving unknown, limit use.

BRAND	ACCEPTABLE		NOT RECOMMENDED
	With added acceptable ingredients and 30% or less calories from fat	With added acceptable ingredients greater than 30% fat (but less than 6 g fat per serving) or fat/serving is unknown (LIMIT USE)	6 or more grams fat per serving or contains added saturated fats
Ragu (Cont'd)	Thick and Hearty: ▲Meat	Thick and Hearty: ▲Mushroom ▲Plain	
Weight Watchers	Spaghetti sauce: ▲Meat ▲Mushroom		

▲ High sodium, 400 mg. or greater per serving.

Kosher

■ **Without added saturated fat, most are high in sodium**
Acceptable choices are listed as those processed without added
saturated fat.

NOT RECOMMENDED

■ **With added saturated fat**
Food choices with added saturated fat are not recommended with the
following exceptions:

- Soups identified with an asterisk (*) indicate that chicken fat
  (a saturated fat) has been added. These soups can be made acceptable if stored in the refrigerator to allow the fat to harden and then
  skimmed before heating.

- Soups identified with a double asterisk (**) contain palm oil in the
  seasoning packet. These soups can be made acceptable if half of a
  bouillon cube is used instead of the seasoning packet.

NOTE

- Most food products in this category do not give nutrition labeling
  information and are therefore evaluated by ingredient labeling alone.

- Although not indicated on the label, most processed kosher foods in
  this section are high in sodium. Sodium symbols are used to indicate
  high (▲) or low (▽) sodium **only** when sodium content is provided on
  the product label. Those products that are not identified with either
  symbol may be either high or low sodium or contain between
  141-399 mg. sodium per serving.

BRAND	ACCEPTABLE	NOT RECOMMENDED
	Without added saturated fat most are high in sodium	With added saturated fat
Carmel Kosher	Soup base chicken style Steak sauce with mushrooms *Strawberry gelatin*	*Imitation chicken flavored fat* Potato pancake and kugel mix *Schmaltz-E-Dige*
Croyden House	Matzo ball and soup mix	*Beef, onion and vegetable instant soup mix* Rice with vermicelli, chicken and beef flavored
Fantastic Foods	★Fantastic falafil mix	
Goodman's	▽Alphabets, enriched egg noodles	Instant onion soup and dip mix Noodleman noodle soup mix
Greenfield's	Egg noodles: ▽•Bowtie ▽•Extra fine ▽•Wide ▽•Enriched egg drop farfel	
Hanover	▲★Chick peas	
Joyva	Sesame crunch	Marble Halvah
Krinos	†Alfonso olives *†Calamata olives* Grape leaves †Tahini *Toursia Giardiniera*	

▲ High sodium, 400 mg. or greater per serving.
▽ Low sodium, 140 mg. or less per serving.
• Contains egg yolks.
† High fat, limit use.
★ High fiber, 3 g. or greater per serving.

BRAND	ACCEPTABLE	NOT RECOMMENDED
	Without added saturated fat most are high in sodium	With added saturated fat

Manischewitz	•Alphabet noodle soup mix, dry
	Bakit seasoned coating
	Borscht and beets
	Condensed barley and mushroom soup
	Condensed tomato soup
	▽Dietetic matzo-thins
	•Egg n' onion matzos
	Fishlets
	Gefilte fish in liquid broth
	Kosher dill pickles
	Low calorie borscht
	Matzo ball mix
	•Matzo ball soup
	•Matzo balls in broth
	Matzo farfel
	▽Matzo meal unsalted
	Minestrone soup mix
	•Noodle soup with vegetables, dry
	Potato kugel mix
	★Split pea soup mix with barley
	Thin salted matzos
	Tomato and mushroom sauce
	Unsalted matzo meal
	•Vegetable soup mix with mushrooms
	Whitefish and pike in jellied broth
		**Bowties noodle soup mix*
		Chicken soup with kreplach
		Chicken soup with matzo balls
		*Condensed chicken soup
		Crackers:
		  Garlic Tams
		  Onion Tams
		  Tam Tam
		  Wheat Tams
		**Lima bean soup mix with barley

▽ Low sodium, 140 mg. or less per serving.
• Contains egg yolks.
* Products containing chicken fat may be acceptable if skimmed before using. Store in refrigerator to allow fat to harden, then skim.
**These soups can be made acceptable if prepared using one half of a bouillon cube instead of the seasoning packet.
★ High fiber, 3 g. or greater per serving.

BRAND	ACCEPTABLE	NOT RECOMMENDED
	Without added saturated fat **most are high in sodium**	**With added saturated fat**
Manischewitz (Cont'd)	▽★Whole wheat matzo cracker with bran Whole wheat matzos	
Mother's	All whitefish in jellied broth ▽Low sodium gefilte fish Old world sweet gefilte fish in jellied broth ▽Unsalted borscht	

Mrs. Weiss	Egg noodles:
	  ▽•Plain (thin and wide)
	  •Rainbow
	  ▽•Spinach
	•Kluski egg noodle	

Rokeach	★*Condensed barley and bean soup* Old Vienna gefilte fish: Sweet recipe *Redi-jellied broth* ★•Split pea and egg barley soup Tomato sauce with mushroom	Dutch pretzels
Streit's	Moonstrips matzos: Onion flavored *Strawberry flavored gel* Unsalted matzos	**Egg drop soup mix* Fried rice soup mix
Telma	★*Fallafel mix* Hommous Tehina sauce	
Wolf's	★Kasha, roasted buckwheat kernels	

▽ Low sodium, 140 mg. or less per serving.
★ High fiber, 3 g. or greater per serving.
• Contains egg yolks.
**These soups can be made acceptable if prepared using one half of a bouillon cube instead of the seasoning packet.

Mexican

Without added saturated fat, may be high in total fat, may be high in sodium

Acceptable choices are listed as those processed without added saturated fat; however, some may be high in total fat.

NOT RECOMMENDED

With added saturated fat

Unacceptable choices are those that have added saturated fat.

NOTE

- Most food products in this category do not provide nutrition labeling information and are therefore evaluated by ingredient labeling alone. As a general rule, all fried foods such as taco shells or tortilla chips are high in fat and should be eaten in limited amounts.

- Although usually not indicated on the food label, most processed Mexican foods are high in sodium. Sodium symbols are used to indicate high (▲) or low (▽) sodium **only** when sodium content is provided on the product label. Those products that are not identified with either symbol may be either high or low sodium or contain between 141-399 mg. sodium per serving.

BRAND	ACCEPTABLE	NOT RECOMMENDED
	Without added saturated fat **may be high in total fat** **may be high in sodium**	**With added saturated fat**

Aztec	Corn tortillas
	Flour tortillas
	Light and Crispy:
	   ▽†Salad shells
	   ▽Taco shells	

Bush's Best	★Chili hot beans	
Camacho	★Chili hot beans Corn tortillas Nacho corn chips	Flour tortillas
Casa Fiesta		Refried beans
ChiChi's	Picante sauce Salsa	
Chico		*Nacho cheese sauce*
Derby		*Beef tamales with sauce*
Don Marcos	▽Corn tortillas	Flour tortillas
El Ebro		Black beans: Cuban style
El Rio	Beef taco filling Chili con carne ★Garbanzo beans Green chopped chilis Honey-Cins *Jalapeño strips nachos*	Hot tamales with chili sauce Mexican cheese dip Nacho cheese sauce

▽ Low sodium, 140 mg. or less per serving.
† High fat, limit use.
★ High fiber, 3 g. or greater per serving.

BRAND	ACCEPTABLE	NOT RECOMMENDED
	Without added saturated fat may be high in total fat may be high in sodium	With added saturated fat
El Rio (Cont'd)	★Mexican beans Nacho-O's ★Refried beans Taco nacho chip dip *Taco seasoning* Tomato and jalapeño peppers Whole jalapeños	
Enrico's	Salsa and taco salsa	
Fontova	Beef tamales Beef tamales with mole sauce Corn tortillas Flour tortillas	Refried beans with mole sauce
French's	Taco seasoning	
Frito Lay	Salsa	Bean dip Jalapeño and cheddar cheese dip
Hain	Hot bean dip Onion bean dip	
Hanover	★Chick peas	
Hodgson Mills	"All Natural" jalapeño (Mexican style) corn bread mix	Jalapeño cornbread mix
Hot Cha Cha	▽Salsa ▽Texas salsa	
Kroger	*Hot peppers* Picante sauce Taco sauce *Taco seasoning mix*	Cheese dip Refried beans Taco shells

▽ Low sodium, 140 mg. or less per serving.
★ High fiber, 3 g. or greater per serving.

BRAND	ACCEPTABLE	NOT RECOMMENDED
	Without added saturated fat may be high in total fat may be high in sodium	With added saturated fat
La Cocina		*Nacho cheese sauce*
La Preferida	★Garbanzos/chick peas Guava nectar Jalapeño nacho slices Jalapeño mustard Jalapeño salsa Louisiana hot sauce Mango nectar Mexicana salsa Mole Papaya nectar with pineapple juice Picante sauce ★Pinto beans ★Pinto beans and jalapeños Ranchero salsa *Salsa picosa* Sliced and pickled jalapeño peppers Sport peppers Taco sauce	Enchilada sauce Refried beans: 　Ranchero style 　Regular 　With sausage
La Victoria	▽Chili dip Enchilada sauce ▽Low sodium salsa Marinated jalapeño peppers Nacho jalapeños ★Refried beans ▽Salsa brava	

▽ Low sodium, 140 mg. or less per serving.
★ High fiber, 3 g. or greater per serving.

BRAND	ACCEPTABLE	NOT RECOMMENDED
	Without added saturated fat may be high in total fat may be high in sodium	With added saturated fat
La Victoria (Cont'd)	▽Salsa casera Salsa jalapeña ▽Salsa picante ▽Salsa Victoria Taco sauce	
Lawry's	Burrito seasoning mix *Chunky taco sauce* Fajitas seasoning Guacamole seasoning blend Taco seasoning	

Little Bear Organic Foods	Organic blue corn taco shells
	Refried beans:
	  ▽★No salt added
	  ★Regular	

McCormick	Enchilada sauce mix Taco seasoning mix	Nacho cheese sauce mix

Old El Paso	*Beef taco filling*
	Burrito dinner
	Mexican rice
	▽Nachips
	Pickled jalapeño slices
	Salsa:
	  Hot picante
	  Medium picante
		Enchilada sauce
		Jalapeño bean dip
		Mexican cheese dip
		Refried beans:
		  Regular
		  with Cheese
		  with Sausage

▽ Low sodium, 140 mg. or less per serving.
★ High fiber, 3 g. or greater per serving.

BRAND	ACCEPTABLE	NOT RECOMMENDED
	Without added saturated fat may be high in total fat may be high in sodium	With added saturated fat
Old El Paso (Cont'd)	Salsa (Cont'd): Mild picante Taco dinner Taco sauce (mild, hot) Taco seasoning mix Taco shells Tomatoes and green chili ▽Tostaco shells	

Ortega	*Chicken seasoning mix*
	★Refried beans
	Salsa:
	  Hot
	  Medium
	  Mild
	Taco dinner
	Taco sauce
	Taco seasoning mix
	▽Taco shells
	▽Tostada shells	

Pace	▽Picante sauce	
Pancho Villa	*Taco dinner* ▽Taco shells ▽Tostada shells	Cheddar cheese sauce
Pepitos	Chunky salsa	

▽ Low sodium, 140 mg. or less per serving.
★ High fiber, 3 g. or greater per serving.

BRAND	ACCEPTABLE	NOT RECOMMENDED
	Without added saturated fat may be high in total fat may be high in sodium	With added saturated fat
Piñata	*Corn tortillas* *Flour tortillas*	
Quaker	▽Corn tortilla mix (Masa harina)	
Ro-tel	Diced tomatoes with green chiles Whole tomatoes with green chiles	
Snack Time	Jalapeño bean dip Taco Mexican dip	Delux cheddar cheese dip Nacho cheese dip
Tobasco	Picante sauce	
Trappey's	Tobasco peppers in vinegar Whole jalapeño peppers	
Vigo	Mexican style rice dinner: Chicken flavored Yellow rice dinner	
Williams	Taco seasoning	Nacho cheese sauce mix
Ye Olde Tyme	Jalapeño corn bread mix *Sopaipilla mix*	

▽ Low sodium, 140 mg. or less per serving.

Oriental

ACCEPTABLE

Without added saturated fat, may be high in sodium
Acceptable choices are listed as those processed without added saturated fat.

NOT RECOMMENDED

With added saturated fat or batter mix designed only for deep fat frying
Products with added saturated fat or those designed to be used only for deep fat frying are not recommended.

NOTE

- Most food products in this category do not give nutrition labeling information and are therefore evaluated by ingredient labeling alone.

- Sodium information is unavailable for most foods in this section. Processed Oriental foods are usually high in sodium. Sodium symbols are used to indicate high (▲) or low (▽) sodium **only** when sodium content is provided on the product label. Those products that are not identified with either symbol may be either high or low sodium or contain between 141-399 mg. sodium per serving.

BRAND	ACCEPTABLE	NOT RECOMMENDED
	Without added saturated fat may be high in sodium	With added saturated fat or batter mix designed only for deep fat frying
All brands	Rice: All types Water chestnuts (canned)	
Angostura	Soy sauce: ▽62% less sodium	
Aristocrat	*Sweet and sour sauce*	
Calbee	†Shrimp flavored chips	
Charlotte Charles	Great Impressions sweet and sour sauce	

Chico San	Mini rice cakes:
	  ▽All flavors
	Popcorn cakes:
	  ▽All flavors
	Rice cakes:
	  ▽All flavors	

China Boy	†Chow mein noodles	
Dynasty	Black bean sauce Stir-fry vegetables	*Oriental style chicken stock Tempura batter mix
Empress	Bamboo shoots	
Erewhon	†Sesame tahini	
Far East	Teriyaki sauce	
Hapi	Mandarin orange float drink	
Hime	Noodles	

▽ Low sodium, 140 mg. or less per serving.
† High fat, limit use.
* Some soups are listed in the "not recommended" column simply because they have added poultry or beef fat. Broth based soups can be made acceptable if they are stored in the refrigerator allowing the fat to harden and then skimmed before heating.

BRAND	ACCEPTABLE	NOT RECOMMENDED
	Without added saturated fat may be high in sodium	With added saturated fat or batter mix designed only for deep fat frying
House of Tsang	Lemon luau †Wok oil	Mabo tofu sauce
IWAI	†Sesame chili oil	
Japanfood	Oriental style noodle	
JFC International	Yoshimure: Rice cracker	

KA-ME	Baby corn
	Black bean sauce
	Chili bits
	†Chili oil
	Chinese cooking rice wine
	Chinese light soy sauce
	Chinese style hot mustard
	Dried black mushrooms
	Duck sauce
	Fermented black beans
	Fish sauce
	Five spice powder
	Five spice sauce and marinade
	Ginger slices
	Hoisin sauce
	Hot chili sauce with garlic
	Hot mustard sauce
	Japanese teriyaki sauce
	Kumquat
	Lychees (canned)
		Instant wonton soup:
		  Chicken
		  Pork
		KA-ME ramen:
		  Beef
		  Chicken
		  Mushroom flavored
		  Pork
		  Shrimp
		KA-ME wonton:
		  Chicken
		  Pork
		Rice crunch crackers:
		  Cheese
		Szechuan sauce
		Tempura batter mix

† High fat, limit use.

BRAND	ACCEPTABLE	NOT RECOMMENDED
	Without added saturated fat may be high in sodium	With added saturated fat or batter mix designed only for deep fat frying

KA-ME (Cont'd)	Mandarine orange sauce
	▲Mild soy sauce, salt reduced
	Noodles:
	    Chinese lo mein
	    Chinese plain
	    Japanese buckwheat
	    Japanese somen
	    Japanese thick
	    Rice sticks (Py Mai Fun)
	    Sai fun bean threads (cellophane noodles)
	    Wide LoMan noodle
	Oyster flavor sauce
	Papaya chunks in light syrup
	Party mix
	Plum sauce
	Rice crunch crackers:
	    ▽Onion
	    ▽Plain
	    ▽Sesame
	Rice snacks
	Rice wine vinegar
	†Sesame oil
	▽†Sesame tempura oil
	Sliced mango
	Smoked baby clams
	Smoked oysters	

† High fat, limit use.
▲ High sodium, 400 mg. or greater per serving.
▽ Low sodium, 140 mg. or less per serving.

BRAND	ACCEPTABLE	NOT RECOMMENDED
	Without added saturated fat may be high in sodium	With added saturated fat or batter mix designed only for deep fat frying
KA-ME (Cont'd)	*Smoked shrimp* Soy sauce (dark) *Star anise* Stir fry corn Stir fry sauce Straw mushrooms ▲Tamari (soy bean sauce) Tiger lily buds *Tow-Fu (canned)*	
Kikkoman	Chinese style seafood soup mix: Shrimp flavor Instant shiro-miso soup ▽Lite soy sauce Marinade mix for meat Soy sauce ▽Steak sauce ▽Stir fry sauce Stir-fry seasoning mix ▽Sukiyaki sauce Sweet and sour mix ▽Sweet and sour sauce Sweet cooking rice wine Tempura sauce ▽Teriyaki marinade ▽Tofu ▽Tonkatsu sauce	Chow mein seasoning mix Fried rice seasoning mix Teriyaki sauce mix

▲ High sodium, 400 mg. or greater per serving.
▽ Low sodium, 140 mg. or less per serving.

BRAND	ACCEPTABLE	NOT RECOMMENDED
	Without added saturated fat may be high in sodium	With added saturated fat or batter mix designed only for deep fat frying
Kroger	Ramen: ▲Beef flavor ▲Chicken flavor ▲Oriental flavor ▲Pork flavor Soy sauce	
La Choy	▽Bean sprouts ▲Chinese fried rice Chop Suey vegetables ▲Chow Mein beef ▲Chow Mein beef mix †Chow Mein noodles †Crispy wide noodles ▽Fancy mixed vegetables Fortune cookies ▽Lite soy sauce ▲Oriental vegetables and sauce mix for pepper steak dinner ▲†Rice noodles ▲Soy sauce (1029 mg sodium/Tbsp.) ▲Sweet and sour chicken ▲*Sweet and sour pork, fruit and vegetables* Sweet and sour sauce	Chicken teriyaki Chow Mein chicken Chow Mein chicken mix Chow Mein shrimp
Lan Chi	Chili paste and garlic	

▲ High sodium, 400 mg. or greater per serving.
▽ Low sodium, 140 mg. or less per serving.
† High fat, limit use.

BRAND	ACCEPTABLE	NOT RECOMMENDED
	Without added saturated fat may be high in sodium	With added saturated fat or batter mix designed only for deep fat frying

Lawry's	Special Edition:
	  Stir-fry sauce
	  Sweet 'n sour
	Teriyaki marinade	

Lea and Perrins	Secret of the Orient:
	  Hong Kong sweet and sour seasoning
	  Mandarin fried rice seasoning
	  Shanghai stir-fry vegetable seasoning
	  Szechuan chicken seasoning	

Maruchan		Instant lunch:
		  Vegetable beef flavor
		Wonton soup mix:
		  Beef flavor
		  Vegetable pork flavor

Mochiko	Sweet rice flour	
Myojo shin – Chukazanmai		Japanese style noodles with soup stock: All flavors

Nissin	Cup o' Noodle oriental noodle soup:
	  with Shrimp
	Alimentary paste
		Cup o'Noodle oriental noodle soup:
		  *Beef flavor
		  *Chicken flavor
		  *Chicken mushroom flavor

Reese	Baby corn Sweet 'n tart sauce	

* Some soups are listed in the "not recommended" column simply because they have added poultry or beef fat. Broth based soups can be made acceptable if they are stored in the refrigerator allowing the fat to harden and then skimmed before heating.

BRAND	ACCEPTABLE	NOT RECOMMENDED
	Without added saturated fat may be high in sodium	**With added saturated fat or batter mix designed only for deep fat frying**
Roger Hong's	Chinese BBQ sauce ▽†Special blend oil Stir-fry sauce Teriyaki sauce	

S and B – Sun Bird	Oriental seasoning mix:
	    Beef and broccoli
	    Chop suey
	    Chow mein
	    Fried rice
	    Stir fry
	Wasabi (Japanese horseradish)	

Sanwa	Sanwa Ramen Pride oriental noodles and:
	    ▲Beef flavor packet
	    ▲Chicken flavor packet
	    ▲Mushroom flavor packet
	    ▲Pork flavor packet
	    ▲Shrimp flavor packet	

Sapporo Ichiban		Japanese style noodles with fried bean curd and soup base:
		    Miso flavor
		    Regular

Streit's	Chow Mein:
	    Mushroom
	    Vegetable	

▲ High sodium, 400 mg. or greater per serving.
▽ Low sodium, 140 mg. or less per serving.
† High fat, limit use.

BRAND	ACCEPTABLE	NOT RECOMMENDED
	Without added saturated fat may be high in sodium	With added saturated fat or batter mix designed only for deep fat frying
Sushi Chef	▽*Reduced sodium dark soy sauce*	
Ty Ling		Ramen: 　All flavors
UMEYA	Fortune cookies	
Wel-Pac	Dried seaweed (musubi nori) Green bamboo shoots Mung beans	

▽ Low sodium, 140 mg. or less per serving.

FATS AND OILS

This section contains listings for the following food categories:

◇ Fats and Oils
◇ Margarine
◇ Peanut Butter
◇ Salad Dressings (Prepared)
◇ Salad Dressings (Dry)

Fat is an essential nutrient, but one that is needed in only very small amounts. Fats in food carry vitamins A, D, E, and K into the body, help insulate the body against heat loss and protect vital organs from injury.

Although light in weight, fat is very dense in calories. In fact, the caloric content of one gram of fat is greater than 2 times the caloric content of one gram of carbohydrate or protein. Hence, it is important to limit all fats in the diet so that not more than 30% of total daily calories come from fat. Choosing appropriate types of fat is just as important as monitoring the amount of fat you eat. Although all vegetable fats are cholesterol-free, some still contain saturated fat, which is the key substance that contributes to elevated cholesterol. Use the following table to help guide you in your fat selections.

Fat type and effect on cholesterol levels

Saturated	Monounsaturated	Polyunsaturated
Elevates cholesterol	Lowers cholesterol	Lowers cholesterol

RECOMMENDATIONS

Avoid Use	Moderate Use	Limit Use
Animal Fats bacon beef fat chicken fat fatty meats lamb fat lard salt pork **Dairy Products** butter cheese cream ice cream 2% milk whole milk **Nuts** coconut **Tropical Oils or Shortenings** cocoa butter coconut palm palm kernel **Unspecified**** vegetable oils, hardened oils or shortenings	**Vegetable Oils** avocado canola high oleic safflower high oleic sunflower olive peanut **Fruit** avocado olives **Nuts***** acorns almonds beechnuts cashews chestnuts filberts or hazelnuts hickory nuts macadamia nuts peanuts pecans pistachios	**Vegetable Oils** corn safflower sesame soybean sunflower **Soft Margarines or Mayonnaise*** with P:S ratio of $\geqslant$2:1 **Nuts****** Brazil nuts butternuts pine nuts walnuts **Seeds** sesame sunflower pumpkin

*Mayonnaise contains egg yolks, however, the amount of cholesterol provided is very minimal, usually less than 10 mg. per serving.

**The source of oil is unknown, therefore treat them as if they were saturated fats.

***The predominant fat in these nuts is monounsaturated.

****The predominant fat in these nuts is polyunsaturated.

Fats and Oils

▨ Monounsaturated oils (MODERATE USE)

Fats and oils listed in this category are the richest sources of mono-unsaturated fat which is a type of fat known to lower LDL cholesterol levels. As discussed on p. 18, the American Heart Association recommends that the greatest proportion of fat in the diet come from monounsaturated sources.

▨ Polyunsaturated oils (LIMIT USE)

Fats and oils listed in this category are the richest sources of polyunsaturated fat. Polyunsaturated fat is known to lower LDL cholesterol levels, but may also lower HDL cholesterol. Although small amounts of these fats are important for health, it is recommended that they be limited to no more than 10% of total calories.

▨ Hydrogenated oils (LIMIT USE)

Shortenings made from hydrogenated acceptable oils should be used in very limited amounts. The saturated fat content of shortenings is at least $1\frac{1}{2}$ times greater than that of its liquid oil counterpart. In addition, their content of trans fatty acids is substantially higher (see page 15 for discussion of negative effects of trans fatty acids). Hydrogenated oils (shortenings) are traditionally used in commercially prepared foods such as breads, crackers and dry mixes.

NOT RECOMMENDED

▨ Saturated fats

Products high in saturated fats are not recommended.

NOTE

- Oils and shortenings contain **no** sodium. Products not marked with the low sodium symbol (▽) are those that do not list nutrition information on their labels.

BRAND	ACCEPTABLE			NOT RECOMMENDED
	Monounsaturated Oils (MODERATE USE)	Polyunsaturated Oils (LIMIT USE)	Hydrogenated Oils (LIMIT USE)	Saturated Fats
OILS:				
All brands	Avocado oil Canola oil High oleic safflower High oleic sunflower Olive oil Peanut oil	Corn oil Safflower oil Sesame oil Soybean oil Sunflower oil		
Avo Co	Avocado oil			
Bertolli	▽Olive oil			
Cost Cutter		Cost Cutter vegetable oil (soybean)		
Crisco		▽Corn oil ▽Crisco pure vegetable oil (soybean)		
Eden	▽Olive oil			
Filippo Berio	▽Olive oil			
Gift of Bran	▽Rice bran oil			
Hain	▽Hain high oleic safflower oil Hain high oleic sunflower oil ▽Hain olive oil ▽Hain peanut oil	▽Hain cold pressed all-blended oil ▽Hain corn oil ▽Hain safflower oil ▽Hain sesame oil ▽Hain soy oil ▽Hain sunflower oil		
Hollywood	▽Canola oil	▽100% pure safflower oil		

▽ Low sodium, 140 mg. or less per serving.

BRAND	ACCEPTABLE			NOT RECOMMENDED
	Monounsaturated Oils (MODERATE USE)	Polyunsaturated Oils (LIMIT USE)	Hydrogenated Oils (LIMIT USE)	Saturated Fats
International Bazaar	▽Olive oil			
Iowa Country Store				Iowa Country Store coconut oil
Italica	▽Olive oil			
Kroger	▽Canola oil	▽Kroger 100% all natural pure vegetable oil (soybean) ▽Kroger 100% sunflower oil ▽Kroger pure corn oil		
Loriva	▽Canola oil ▽Peanut oil	▽Sesame oil		
Mazola		▽Mazola 100% pure corn oil		
Old Monk	Olive oil			
Planters	▽100% pure peanut oil			
Pompeian	▽Olive oil			
Progresso	Olive oil			
Puritan	▽Puritan 100% pure vegetable oil (canola)			
Spectrum Naturals	Canola oil High oleic safflower oil ▽Unrefined high oleic sunflower oil			

▽ Low sodium, 140 mg. or less per serving.

Brand	Acceptable			Not Recommended
	Monounsaturated Oils (MODERATE USE)	Polyunsaturated Oils (LIMIT USE)	Hydrogenated Oils (LIMIT USE)	Saturated Fats
Wesson		▽Corn oil ▽Sunlite sunflower oil ▽Vegetable oil, light and natural (soybean) ▽Wesson vegetable oil (soybean)		
POPCORN OILS:				
Orville Redenbacher		Orville Redenbacher's gourmet popcorn oil: ▽Buttery flavor (soybean)		
SHORTENING:				
Cost Cutter				*Cost Cutter precreamed shortening*
Crisco			All vegetable shortening ▽Crisco butter flavor all vegetable shortening	
Kroger			▽Kroger all vegetable shortening	Kroger butter flavor all vegetable shortening
SPRAYS:				
Baker's Joy		▽Baker's Joy (baking spray)		
Kroger		▽Buttery cooking spray		No stick cooking spray
Mazola		▽No stick corn oil cooking spray		

▽ Low sodium, 140 mg. or less per serving.

BRAND	ACCEPTABLE			NOT RECOMMENDED
	Monounsaturated Oils (MODERATE USE)	Polyunsaturated Oils (LIMIT USE)	Hydrogenated Oils (LIMIT USE)	Saturated Fats
Pam	▽Pam no stick cooking spray with olive oil	▽Pam no stick butter flavor cooking spray ▽Pam no stick cooking spray		
Weight Watchers		▽Popcorn spray ▽Weight Watchers buttery spray ▽Weight Watchers cooking spray		
LARDS:				
Armour				Armour lard
Bob Evans Country Kitchen				*Bob Evans Country Kitchen brand lard*

▽ Low sodium, 140 mg. or less per serving.

Margarine

ACCEPTABLE

■ **1 gram or less saturated fat per Tbsp. (LIMIT USE)**
These margarines contain the least amount of saturated fat per one table-spoon serving. Although the preferred choice, remember that all margarines are approximately 99% fat and should be consumed in limited quantities.

■ **2 grams or less saturated fat per Tbsp. (LIMIT USE)**
These margarines are higher in saturated fat per serving than those listed in the first category. Because they contain greater amounts of hydroge-nated oils, they are most likely higher in trans fatty acids. Limited intake is recommended.

NOT RECOMMENDED

■ **Greater than 2 grams saturated fat or saturated fat content unknown**
Margarines with a saturated fat content greater than 2 grams per serving are not recommended.

NOTE

- The American Heart Association recommends selecting margarines with a liquid oil listed as the first ingredient.

- Some products listed in the acceptable categories contain butter or cream in varying amounts and are identified with an asterisk (*). These marga-rines or butter blends may contain higher amounts of individual saturated fatty acids that are known to have cholesterol elevating properties. For this reason, we recommend prudent use especially by those individuals with documented coronary heart disease or those who have elevated serum cholesterol.

- Most margarine contains approximately 100 mg. sodium per one table-spoon serving. Sodium symbols are used to indicate high (▲) or low (▽) sodium **only** when sodium content is provided on the product label. Those products that are not identified with either symbol may be either high or low sodium or contain between 141-399 mg. sodium per serving.

BRAND	ACCEPTABLE		NOT RECOMMENDED
	1 gram or less saturated fat per Tbsp. (LIMIT USE)	2 grams or less saturated fat per Tbsp. (LIMIT USE)	Greater than 2 grams saturated fat or saturated fat content unknown
"I Can't Believe It's Not Butter"		▽*Soft margarine (tub) ▽*Squeeze margarine ▽*Stick margarine	
Blue Bonnet	▽48% vegetable oil spread	▽75% vegetable oil spread ▽*Blue Bonnet Butter Blend ▽Blue Bonnet margarine stick ▽Blue Bonnet soft margarine	
Cost Cutter	▽Cost Cutter spread	▽Cost Cutter corn oil margarine ▽Cost Cutter margarine	
Fleischmann's	▽Fleischmann's extra light corn oil ▽Fleischmann's squeeze margarine	▽100% corn oil margarine (stick) ▽Fleischmann's light corn oil spread (stick, tub) ▽Fleischmann's sweet unsalted (stick) ▽Soft Fleischmann's margarine	
Hain		Hain rich in liquid safflower oil margarine Hain rich in liquid soft safflower oil margarine ▽Hain rich in liquid unsalted safflower oil margarine	
Imperial	▽*A la Mode, vegetable oil spread with sweet cream ▽Diet Imperial reduced calorie margarine		Imperial margarine Imperial soft margarine Light Imperial
Kraft	▽*Kraft Touch of Butter		

▽ Low sodium, 140 mg. or less per serving.
* Product contains butter or cream.

BRAND	ACCEPTABLE		NOT RECOMMENDED
	1 gram or less saturated fat per Tbsp. (LIMIT USE)	2 grams or less saturated fat per Tbsp. (LIMIT USE)	Greater than 2 grams saturated fat or saturated fat content unknown
Kroger	▽Kroger lite spread	▽Kroger corn oil margarine ▽Kroger soft spread margarine ▽Stick margarine	
Land O Lakes			Country Morning blend Country Morning blend light and real butter (tub) Country Morning blend light and real butter (stick) Country Morning blend unsalted margarine Land O Lakes margarine Lightly salted spread with sweet cream Lightly salted spread with sweet cream (stick)
Mar-Parv			Kosher and Parve Margarine
Mazola	▽Light corn oil spread	▽Premium margarine sticks	
NUCOA	Heartbeat spread: 　▽20% corn oil		
Parkay	▽Gold spread ▽Parkay spread	▽Parkay margarine ▽Soft Parkay margarine ▽Squeeze Parkay margarine	

▽ Low sodium, 140 mg. or less per serving.

BRAND	ACCEPTABLE		NOT RECOMMENDED
	1 gram or less saturated fat per Tbsp. (LIMIT USE)	2 grams or less saturated fat per Tbsp. (LIMIT USE)	Greater than 2 grams saturated fat or saturated fat content unknown
Promise	▽Promise 68% vegetable oil spread (tub) ▽Promise extra light 40% vegetable oil spread (tub) ▽*Promise light 53% vegetable oil spread (tub)*	▽Promise 68% vegetable oil spread (sticks)	
Shedd's	▽100% corn oil Country Crock ▽Shedd's Spread Country Crock squeezable ▽Shedd's Spread Country Crock	▽Shedd's Spread Country Crock classic quarters Willow Run soybean margarine	
Tree of Life		▽Canola-Soy margarine	
Weight Watchers	Light spread: ▽40% vegetable oil ▽Reduced calorie margarine, unsalted ▽Reduced calorie margarine		
BUTTER SUBSTITUTES:			
Butter Buds	▽*Butter mix ▽*Shaker jar		

Molly McButter	Natural Sprinkles:
	  ▽*Butter flavor
	  ▽*Cheese flavor
	  *Sour cream flavor		

▽ Low sodium, 140 mg. or less per serving.
* Product contains butter or cream.

Peanut Butter

ACCEPTABLE

■ **Without added saturated fat (LIMIT USE)**
Acceptable food choices are those products that are made from ground peanuts without added saturated fats.

NOT RECOMMENDED

■ **With added saturated fat (unspecified hardened oils)**
Peanut butter that contains unspecified hardened vegetable oils are not recommended because the source of the oil is unknown.

NOTE

- The sodium content of most peanut butter ranges between 125-180 mg. per 2 Tbsp. serving. Sodium symbols are used to indicate high (▲) or low (▽) sodium **only** when sodium content is provided on the product label. Those products that are not identified with either symbol may be either high or low sodium or contain between 141-399 mg. sodium per serving.

BRAND	ACCEPTABLE	NOT RECOMMENDED
	Without added Saturated Fat (LIMIT USE)	With added Saturated Fat (Unspecified hardened Oils)
Cost Cutter		Creamy peanut butter
Deaf Smith	Arrowhead Mills: ▽Peanut butter	
Erewhon	Peanut butter: ▽Chunky unsalted ▽Creamy unsalted	
Estee		Low sodium peanut butter
Jif		Peanut butter: Creamy Extra crunchy
Kroger	▽Natural old fashioned peanut butter Nutty-ER, 100% peanut butter	Peanut butter: Creamy Super crunchy
Peter Pan		Peanut butter
Skippy		Peanut butter: Creamy Super chunky
Smucker's	▽Goober Grape—peanut butter and grape jelly ▽Natural peanut butter	
Velvet		Peanut butter: Super creamy Super crunchy

▽ Low sodium, 140 mg. or less per serving.

Salad Dressings (Prepared)

ACCEPTABLE

■ **No oil or less than 1 gram fat per Tbsp. (may be partially hydrogenated)**
These dressings are preferred choices because they contain no added fat or are very low in fat.

■ **Acceptable oils (LIMIT USE)**
Most regular dressings are made with polyunsaturated oils. Because salad dressings are high in fat, their intake should be limited. Those dressings containing monounsaturated fat (i.e., olive and canola oil) are preferred.

■ **Acceptable partially hydrogenated oils (LIMIT USE)**
These salad dressings and/or mayonnaise are also acceptable but should be limited because they are high in fat. Although some of these products contain egg yolks, they provide very little cholesterol per serving (e.g., 5-10 mg. per Tbsp.). These products should be limited because of their fat content, **not** simply because they contain egg yolks.

NOT RECOMMENDED

■ **With added saturated fat**
Salad dressings with added saturated fat are not recommended.

NOTE

■ Buttermilk is less than 1% butterfat and is therefore considered an acceptable ingredient.

■ The approximate sodium content of regular salad dressings is 120 mg. per 1 Tbsp. serving. Sodium symbols are used to indicate high (▲) or low (▽) sodium **only** when sodium content is provided on the product label. Those products that are not identified with either symbol may be either high or low sodium or contain between 141-399 mg. sodium per serving.

BRAND	ACCEPTABLE			NOT RECOMMENDED
	No oil or less than 1 g. fat per Tbsp. (may be partially hydrogenated)	Acceptable oils (LIMIT USE)	Acceptable partially hydrogenated oils (LIMIT USE)	With added saturated fat
Bonique		*Bonique red wine vinegar and oil dressing*		
Bright Day		▽Bright Day cholesterol free dressing		
Charlotte Charles		Great Impressions poppy seed dressing		
Christie's		Christie's Greek salad dressing		
Dia-Mel		•Dia-Mel mayonnaise		
El Molino	El Molino Herbal Secrets: ▽Creamy Italian all natural dressing ▽French style all natural dressing ▽Herbs and spice all natural dressing ▽Italian dressing ▽Vinaigrette all natural dressing			
Estee	Estee: ▽Blue cheese dressing ▽Creamy French dressing	Estee: ▽•Reduced calorie mayonnaise		

▽ Low sodium, 140 mg. or less per serving.
• Contains egg yolks.

BRAND	ACCEPTABLE			NOT RECOMMENDED
	No oil or less than 1 g. fat per Tbsp. (may be partially hydrogenated)	Acceptable oils (LIMIT USE)	Acceptable partially hydrogenated oils (LIMIT USE)	With added saturated fat
Estee (Cont'd)	Estee (Cont'd): ▽Creamy Italian dressing ▽Red wine vinegar dressing ▽•Thousand island dressing ▽Zesty Italian dressing			
Featherweight	Featherweight Healthy Recipes: ▽Creamy cucumber dressing ▽French style dressing ▽Red wine and vinegar dressing ▽Zesty tomato	Featherweight: ▽•Imitation mayonnaise •Imitation French dressing		
Grecian Dressing Enterprises, Inc.		Authentic garlic dressing Authentic Greek dressing		
Hain		Hain: ▽Eggless imitation mayonnaise ▽Eggless mayonnaise ▽•Light mayonnaise ▽•Safflower mayonnaise		Hain Natural Classics: Poppyseed rancher's dressing Hain Naturals: Creamy Caesar Garlic and sour cream dressing

▽ Low sodium, 140 mg. or less per serving.
• Contains egg yolks

BRAND	ACCEPTABLE			NOT RECOMMENDED
	No oil or less than 1 g. fat per Tbsp. (may be partially hydrogenated)	Acceptable oils (LIMIT USE)	Acceptable partially hydrogenated oils (LIMIT USE)	With added saturated fat
Hain (Cont'd)		Hain (Cont'd): ▽•*Unsalted real mayonnaise* Hain Natural Classics: Dijon vinaigrette Hain Naturals: ▽Creamy French dressing *Creamy Italian* •Cucumber dill ▽•Thousand island		Hain Naturals (Cont'd): Old fashioned buttermilk
Hellman's			Hellman's: ▽•Light reduced calorie mayonnaise ▽•Real mayonnaise	
Henri's		▽Henri's 90% fat free private blend Tas-Tee reduced calorie dressing ▽Original recipe private blend Tas-Tee dressing		
Herb Magic	Herb Magic reduced calorie dressing: ▽Creamy cucumber ▽Italian ▽Sweet and sour Vinaigrette			

▽ Low sodium, 140 mg. or less per serving.
• Contains egg yolks.

BRAND	ACCEPTABLE			NOT RECOMMENDED
	No oil or less than 1 g. fat per Tbsp. (may be partially hydrogenated)	Acceptable oils (LIMIT USE)	Acceptable partially hydrogenated oils (LIMIT USE)	With added saturated fat
Hidden Valley Ranch	Take Heart: ▽Blue cheese ▽French ▽Italian reduced calorie dressing ▽Thousand Island		Hidden Valley Ranch: Italian dressing ▽•Original ranch creamy dressing Hidden Valley Ranch reduced calorie: ▽•Original ranch dressing ▽Ranch Italian dressing Take Heart: ▽Original ranch	Hidden Valley Ranch: Original ranch with bacon
Knott's Berry Farm		Fruit salad dressing		
Kraft	Kraft Free nonfat dressings: ▽Catalina ▽French ▽Italian ▽Ranch ▽Thousand Island Kraft Free nonfat mayonnaise dressing Miracle Whip Free nonfat dressing Oil free Italian dressing	Kraft: Catalina French dressing ▽Catalina reduced calorie dressing ▽Cholesterol free mayonnaise ▽French dressing Golden Caesar dressing ▽•House Italian dressing		Kraft: Bacon and tomato dressing Bacon and tomato reduced calorie dressing *Buttermilk creamy reduced calorie dressing* Buttermilk ranch dressing Chunky blue cheese dressing Creamy cucumber

▽ Low sodium, 140 mg. or less per serving.
• Contains egg yolks.

BRAND	ACCEPTABLE			NOT RECOMMENDED
	No oil or less than 1 g. fat per Tbsp. (may be partially hydrogenated)	Acceptable oils (LIMIT USE)	Acceptable partially hydrogenated oils (LIMIT USE)	With added saturated fat
Kraft (Cont'd)		Kraft (Cont'd): ▽Light cholesterol free mayonnaise ▽Miracle Whip cholesterol free salad dressing •Miracle Whip coleslaw dressing ▽Miracle Whip light salad dressing ▽•Miracle Whip salad dressing Presto Italian dressing ▽•Rancher's choice ranch dressing •Rancher's Choice ranch reduced calorie dressing ▽•Real mayonnaise •Sandwich spread •Thousand island dressing •Thousand island reduced calorie dressing Zesty Italian dressing		Kraft (Cont'd): Creamy cucumber reduced calorie dressing Roka blue cheese dressing

▽ Low sodium, 140 mg. or less per serving.
• Contains egg yolks.

BRAND	ACCEPTABLE			NOT RECOMMENDED
	No oil or less than 1 g. fat per Tbsp. (may be partially hydrogenated)	Acceptable oils (LIMIT USE)	Acceptable partially hydrogenated oils (LIMIT USE)	With added saturated fat
Kraft (Cont'd)		Kraft (Cont'd): Zesty Italian reduced calorie dressing Kraft squeezable dressing: *Catalina French* ▽*French* ▽•*Rancher's Creamy* •*Thousand Island* •*Zesty Italian*		
Kroger	Fat Free dressing: Buttermilk California French ▽French Italian ▽Thousand Island Kroger: Lite Italian reduced calorie dressing	Kroger: ▽Cholesterol free lite mayonnaise ▽Cholesterol free lite salad dressing ▽•Cholesterol free mayonnaise •Coleslaw dressing Creamy buttermilk dressing Creamy Italian dressing French dressing Italian dressing Lite buttermilk reduced calorie dressing		Kroger: Bacon and tomato dressing Chunky blue cheese dressing Creamy buttermilk and bacon dressing Creamy cucumber Green Goddess dressing Lite bacon and tomato reduced calorie dressing Lite blue cheese reduced calorie dressing Lite creamy cucumber reduced calorie dressing *Ranchero dressing*

▽ Low sodium, 140 mg. or less per serving.
• Contains egg yolks.

BRAND	ACCEPTABLE			NOT RECOMMENDED
	No oil or less than 1 g. fat per Tbsp. (may be partially hydrogenated)	Acceptable oils (LIMIT USE)	Acceptable partially hydrogenated oils (LIMIT USE)	With added saturated fat
Kroger (Cont'd)		Kroger (Cont'd): •Lite creamy Italian reduced calorie dressing Lite French style reduced calorie dressing •Lite thousand island reduced calorie dressing Poppyseed dressing ▽•Real mayonnaise Real west dressing Russian dressing ▽•Salad dressing ▽•Sandwich spread Sweet and sour dressing •Thousand island dressing		
Lawry's		Lawry's: Italian with aged parmesan cheese dressing Red wine vinaigrette San Francisco with romano cheese White wine vinaigrette		Lawry's: Caesar dressing

▽ Low sodium, 140 mg. or less per serving.
• Contains egg yolks.

BRAND	ACCEPTABLE			NOT RECOMMENDED
	No oil or less than 1 g. fat per Tbsp. (may be partially hydrogenated)	Acceptable oils (LIMIT USE)	Acceptable partially hydrogenated oils (LIMIT USE)	With added saturated fat
Mack's				Honey poppy seed dressing *Tennessee pepper pot dressing*
Marie's		Marie's: Classic herb vinaigrette dressing •Lite ranch reduced calorie dressing •Lite thousand island dressing •Ranch dressing Red wine vinaigrette dressing		Marie's: Blue cheese dressing Buttermilk spice ranch style dressing Creamy Italian garlic dressing Lite blue cheese dressing Lite Italian garlic reduced calorie dressing *Sour cream and dill dressing* Thousand island dressing
Marzetti		Marzetti: •Light slaw dressing •Potato salad dressing •Slaw dressing •*Southern recipe slaw dressing*		
Medford Farms	Medford Farms: ▽No oil bleu cheese lite dressing ▽No oil chef's lite dressing			

▽ Low sodium, 140 mg. or less per serving.
• Contains egg yolks.

BRAND	ACCEPTABLE			NOT RECOMMENDED
	No oil or less than 1 g. fat per Tbsp. (may be partially hydrogenated)	Acceptable oils (LIMIT USE)	Acceptable partially hydrogenated oils (LIMIT USE)	With added saturated fat
Medford Farms (Cont'd)	Medford Farms (Cont'd): ▽No oil Italian lite dressing ▽No oil vinaigrette dressing			
Milani	Milani dill cooking sauce and marinade	Milani French dressing		
Mullen's		Mullen's: *French dressing* *Imitation French dressing*		
Nasoya		Nasoya Vegi-dressing: ▽Creamy dill ▽Garden herb ▽Italian ▽Sesame garlic ▽Nayonaise		
Newman's Own		Olive oil and vinegar dressing Reduced calorie light Italian dressing		
Old Dutch	Old Dutch sweet-sour dressing			
Parthenon		Greek salad dressing		

▽ Low sodium, 140 mg. or less per serving.
• Contains egg yolks.

BRAND	ACCEPTABLE			NOT RECOMMENDED
	No oil or less than 1 g. fat per Tbsp. (may be partially hydrogenated)	Acceptable oils (LIMIT USE)	Acceptable partially hydrogenated oils (LIMIT USE)	With added saturated fat
Pfeiffer		Pfeiffer ▽•Buttermilk and herbs dressing Italian dressing ▽•Thousand island dressing		
Pritikin	Pritikin: ▽No oil French style dressing ▽No oil Italian dressing ▽No oil ranch dressing and marinade ▽No oil Russian dressing ▽No oil vinaigrette			
Reese				Reese poppy seed dressing
Richard Simmons	Salad spray: Italian Roma cheese	Salad spray: ▽French style		
Robb Ross		Robb Ross red wine vinegar and oil dressing		
Seven Seas		Seven Seas: •Buttermilk recipe creamy ranch dressing	Seven Seas: Creamy bacon dressing	Seven Seas: Artificially flavored creamy bacon dressing *Chunky blue cheese*

▽ Low sodium, 140 mg. or less per serving.
• Contains egg yolks.

BRAND	ACCEPTABLE			NOT RECOMMENDED
	No oil or less than 1 g. fat per Tbsp. (may be partially hydrogenated)	Acceptable oils (LIMIT USE)	Acceptable partially hydrogenated oils (LIMIT USE)	With added saturated fat
Seven Seas (Cont'd)		Seven Seas (Cont'd): ▽•*Buttermilk recipe light dressing* Viva creamy Italian dressing Viva Italian dressing Viva Italian light reduced calorie dressing •Viva ranch dressing		
Spectrum Naturals		▽•Canola mayonnaise ▽Eggless reduced calorie mayonnaise spread ▽*Eggless-low fat mayonnaise*		
Sweet Lite		▽•Sweet Lite reduced calorie mayonnaise		
T. Marzetti's		T. Marzetti's: ▽*Buttermilk vegetable dip and dressing* ▽Crispy celery seed dressing ▽•Dijon honey mustard dip and dressing •Fresh buttermilk ranch dressing		T. Marzetti's: *Bacony style spinach salad* Blue cheese veggie dip Buttermilk blue cheese dressing French blue cheese dressing Lite chunky blue cheese Ranch Veggie dip

▽ Low sodium, 140 mg. or less per serving.
• Contains egg yolks.

BRAND	ACCEPTABLE			NOT RECOMMENDED
	No oil or less than 1 g. fat per Tbsp. (may be partially hydrogenated)	Acceptable oils (LIMIT USE)	Acceptable partially hydrogenated oils (LIMIT USE)	With added saturated fat
T. Marzetti's (Cont'd)		T. Marzetti's (Cont'd): ▽•Homestyle thousand island dressing ▽Honey French dressing ▽•Lite buttermilk ranch •Original slaw dressing		
Weight Watchers	Weight Watchers: Caesar salad dressing ▽•Creamy ranch French style dressing Italian style dressing Tomato vinaigrette dressing	Weight Watchers: ▽Cholesterol free reduced calorie mayonnaise ▽•Reduced calorie mayonnaise ▽Whipped reduced calorie mayonnaise ▽•Whipped reduced calorie salad dressing		
Western		▽Original lite western French dressing Original western French dressing		

▽ Low sodium, 140 mg. or less per serving.
• Contains egg yolks.

BRAND	ACCEPTABLE			NOT RECOMMENDED
	No oil or less than 1 g. fat per Tbsp. (may be partially hydrogenated)	Acceptable oils (LIMIT USE)	Acceptable partially hydrogenated oils (LIMIT USE)	With added saturated fat

Wish-Bone	Wish-Bone:
	  Lite Italian reduced calorie dressing
	  ▽Lite Sweet 'n Spicy French style-reduced calorie dressing
		Wish-Bone:
		  Blended Italian
		  Classic dijon vinaigrette dressing
		  Creamy garlic dressing
		  Italian dressing
		  Olive oil Italian
		  ▽Olive oil vinaigrette dressing
		  Red French dressing
		  Red wine vinaigrette dressing
		  •Robusto Italian dressing
		  ▽Russian dressing
		  Sweet 'n Spicy French dressing
			Wish-Bone:
			  •Lite ranch reduced calorie dressing
			  •Ranch dressing
				Wish-Bone:
				  Blue cheese dressing
				  Lite creamy Italian reduced calorie dressing

▽ Low sodium, 140 mg. or less per serving.
• Contains egg yolks.

Salad Dressings (Dry)

ACCEPTABLE

■ **No oil or less than 1 gram fat per Tbsp., may be partially hydrogenated (LIMIT USE),**

■ **Acceptable oils (LIMIT USE), and**

■ **Acceptable partially hydrogenated oils (LIMIT USE)**

Dressing mixes in all three categories contain no added fat or may have added acceptable unsaturated or partially hydrogenated oils. When mixed at home it is recommended that a monounsaturated oil (e.g., olive, canola, high oleic safflower or high oleic sunflower) be used and that you use 1/4 to 1/3 less oil than called for on the package. Furthermore, should the directions call for mayonnaise or sour cream, it is recommended that you substitute nonfat yogurt, buttermilk or reduced fat mayonnaise to minimize the fat content of the dressing.

NOT RECOMMENDED

■ **With added saturated fat**

Salad dressings with added saturated fat are not recommended.

NOTE

■ The approximate sodium content of dry salad dressings prepared following package direction ranges between 120-190 mg. per 1 Tbsp. serving. Sodium symbols are used to indicate high (▲) or low (▽) sodium **only** when sodium content is provided on the product label. Those products that are not identified with either symbol may be either high or low sodium or contain between 141-399 mg. sodium per serving.

BRAND	ACCEPTABLE			NOT RECOMMENDED
	No oil or less than 1 g. fat per Tbsp. may be partially hydrogenated (LIMIT USE)	Acceptable oils (LIMIT USE)	Acceptable partially hydrogenated oils (LIMIT USE)	With added saturated fat
Estee	▽Creamy French dressing mix ▽•Thousand Island dressing mix ▽Zesty Italian dry mix			
Good Season's	Good Season's salad dressing mix: 　Garlic and herbs 　▽Lemon and herbs 　Mild Italian 　No oil Italian 　▽Zesty Italian		Good Season's salad dressing mix: 　Buttermilk farm style	Good Season's salad dressing mix: 　*Cheese garlic* 　Cheese Italian
Hidden Valley Ranch		Hidden Valley Ranch: 　▽Buttermilk recipe original salad dressing mix 　▽Original party dip		Hidden Valley Ranch: 　Italian salad dressing mix 　Original salad dressing mix 　Reduced calorie original salad dressing mix 　Reduced calorie party dip
Kroger	Kroger Salad Magic dressing mix: 　Classic French 　Garlic and herb 　Italian 　Lite Italian			Kroger Salad Magic dressing mix: 　Buttermilk and bac'n buds 　Buttermilk country style

▽ Low sodium, 140 mg. or less per serving.
• Contains egg yolks.

BRAND	ACCEPTABLE			NOT RECOMMENDED
	No oil or less than 1 g. fat per Tbsp. may be partially hydrogenated (LIMIT USE)	Acceptable oils (LIMIT USE)	Acceptable partially hydrogenated oils (LIMIT USE)	With added saturated fat
Weight Watchers	Weight Watchers dressing mix: ▽Blue cheese Caesar salad Creamy Italian ▽•Creamy ranch French style ▲Italian Thousand Island			

▲ High sodium, greater than 400 mg. per serving.
▽ Low sodium, 140 mg. or less per serving.
• Contains egg yolks.

FROZEN FOODS

This section contains listings with criteria for evaluating the following food categories:

◇ Entrees
◇ Desserts
◇ Vegetables

Frozen foods provide convenient, quick meals for people with busy lifestyles. Although **not** preferred over fresh foods or home prepared meals, these products may be used occasionally if ingredient and nutrient labeling are carefully evaluated. A growing number of frozen food manufacturers are responding to the consumer's demand for lower calorie "lean" food options. Informed consumers should evaluate food products by both the quantity of calories and by the quality of those calories. When evaluating frozen entrees, the amount of fat, as well as sodium should be considered.

Entrees

▨ **30% or less calories from fat, 800 mg. sodium or less (LIMIT USE)**
Acceptable food choices are evaluated according to fat and sodium content. Since frozen entrees are designed to supply approximately one third of a person's daily intake, the food choices deemed acceptable are those that contain 30% or less of their calories from fat and less than or equal to 800 mg. of sodium.

Not Recommended

▨ **Greater than 30% calories from fat, greater than 800 mg. sodium**
Entrees containing greater than 30% calories from fat and/or greater than 800 mg. of sodium are not recommended.

Note

■ Most frozen entrees are high in sodium ranging between 500-1500 mg. per serving. Sodium symbols are used to indicate high (▲) or low (▽) sodium **only** when sodium content is provided on the product label. Those products that are not identified with either symbol may be either high or low sodium or contain between 141-399 mg. sodium per serving.

BRAND	ACCEPTABLE	NOT RECOMMENDED
	30% or less calories from fat 800 mg. sodium or less (LIMIT USE)	Greater than 30% calories from fat greater than 800 mg. sodium
Armour Classics		Lite Beef Stroganoff
Armour Dinner Classic Lite	▲Chicken a la king ▲Steak Diane	Beef stroganoff Chicken burgundy Salisbury steak Sweet and sour chicken
Armour Dinner Classics		Boneless beef short ribs Chicken and noodles Chicken fettucini Chicken mesquite Chicken parmigiana Chicken with wine and mushroom sauce Glazed chicken Salisbury steak Sirloin roast Sirloin tips Swedish meatballs Turkey with dressing and gravy Veal parmigiana Yankee pot roast

Aunt Jemima	▲★•Lite microwave pancakes
	Waffles:
	  Oat bran
		Homestyle breakfast:
		  Four pancakes with three bacon slices
		  Four pancakes with two sausages
		  Scrambled eggs and cheddar cheese with home fried potatoes

▲ High sodium, greater than 400 mg. per serving.
• Contains egg yolks.
★ High fiber, 3 g. or greater per serving.

BRAND	ACCEPTABLE	NOT RECOMMENDED
	30% or less calories from fat 800 mg. sodium or less (LIMIT USE)	Greater than 30% calories from fat greater than 800 mg. sodium

Aunt Jemima (Cont'd)		Homestyle breakfast (Cont'd):
		    Scrambled eggs and sausage with hashed
		        brown potatoes
		    Three french toast wedges with two
		        sausages

Campbell's		Souper Combo:
		    Chicken and stars soup and breaded
		        chicken nuggets
		    Chicken noodle o's and hot dog on a bun
		    Chicken rice soup and vegetable egg rolls
		    Chili with beans and hot dog on a bun
		    Cream of broccoli soup and ham and
		        cheese croissant sandwich
		    Minestrone soup and breaded mozzarella
		        cheese sticks
		    *New England clam chowder and breaded
		        fish sandwich*
		    Tomato soup and grilled cheese sandwich
		    Vegetable soup and cheeseburger

Healthy Choice	▲Beef pepper steak dinner ▲Breast of Turkey ▲Chicken and pasta divan ▲Chicken oriental dinner Chicken parmigiana dinner •Fettucini Alfredo Glazed Chicken	

▲ High Sodium, greater than 400 mg. per serving.
• Contains egg yolks.

BRAND	ACCEPTABLE	NOT RECOMMENDED
	30% or less calories from fat 800 mg. sodium or less (LIMIT USE)	**Greater than 30% calories from fat greater than 800 mg. sodium**
Healthy Choice (Cont'd)	Mesquite chicken dinner ▲*Oriental pepper steak* ▲Salisbury steak dinner ▲Seafood Newburg ▲Shrimp creole dinner Sirloin tips dinner ▲Sole au gratin Sole with lemon butter Sweet and sour chicken dinner	
Kroger	Premium Dinner: 　▲*Sweet and sour chicken*	Premium Dinner: 　Beef sirloin tips 　Chicken a la king 　Chicken parmigiana 　Pepper steak 　Salisbury steak 　Sliced turkey
Lean Pockets	•*Beef and broccoli* •Chicken supreme	Pizza
LeMenu	▲•Breast of chicken ▲Chicken a la king	*3-cheese manicotti* Beef sirloin tips Beef stroganoff Chicken cordon bleu Chicken parmigiana Chopped sirloin beef Ham steak

▲ High sodium, greater than 400 mg. per serving.
• Contains egg yolks.

BRAND	ACCEPTABLE 30% or less calories from fat 800 mg. sodium or less (LIMIT USE)	NOT RECOMMENDED Greater than 30% calories from fat greater than 800 mg. sodium
LeMenu (Cont'd)		Pepper steak Salisbury steak Sliced turkey breast Sweet and sour chicken Veal parmigiana Yankee pot roast
LeMenu — Light Style	▲•Chicken cannelloni ▲Chicken chow mein ▲Chicken dijon ▲Glazed chicken breast ▲Herb roasted chicken ▲•Lasagna and meat sauce ▲Veal marsala	Salisbury steak Turkey divan

Old El Paso		Beef and bean burrito:
		   Hot
		   Medium
		   Mild
		Chimichangas:
		   Beef
		   Chicken
		Enchiladas:
		   Chicken

Stouffer's Dinner Supreme		Baked chicken breast Bar-b-que style chicken

▲ High sodium, greater than 400 mg. per serving.
• Contains egg yolks.

BRAND	ACCEPTABLE	NOT RECOMMENDED
	30% or less calories from fat 800 mg. sodium or less (LIMIT USE)	Greater than 30% calories from fat greater than 800 mg. sodium
Stouffer's Dinner Supreme (Cont'd)		*Beef teriyaki* *Cheese stuffed shells* *Chicken Florentine* Chicken parmigiana *Chicken with supreme sauce* *Fried chicken* *Glazed ham steak* *Homestyle meat loaf* *Roast turkey breast with gravy and dressing* Salisbury steak *Turkey divan* Veal parmigiana
Stouffer's Lean Cuisine	Chicken a l'orange ▲Filet of fish divan French bread pizza: ▲Cheese ▲Sliced turkey breast in mushroom sauce	*Beef and pork cannelloni* Beefsteak ranchero Breast of chicken in herb cream sauce Breast of chicken marsala Breast of chicken parmesan Cheese cannelloni Chicken and vegetables with vermicelli Chicken cacciatore Chicken chow mein Chicken oriental Fiesta chicken Filet of fish florentine

▲ High sodium, greater than 400 mg. per serving.

BRAND	ACCEPTABLE	NOT RECOMMENDED
	30% or less calories from fat 800 mg. sodium or less (LIMIT USE)	**Greater than 30% calories from fat greater than 800 mg. sodium**
Stouffer's Lean Cuisine (Cont'd)		*Filet of fish jardiniere* French bread pizza: Deluxe Pepperoni Sausage Glazed chicken Lasagna with meat and sauce Linguini with clam sauce Meatball stew Oriental beef Rigatoni bake *Salisbury steak* *Shrimp and chicken cantonese* Spaghetti with beef and mushroom sauce Stuffed cabbage *Szechwan beef* Tuna lasagna Turkey dijon Vegetable and pasta mornay with ham Zucchini lasagna
Stouffer's Right Course	▲Beef dijon with pasta and vegetables ▲*Beef ragout with rice pilaf* ▲Chicken Italiano with fettucini and vegetables ▲Chicken tenderloins in barbecue sauce with rice pilaf	

▲ High sodium, greater than 400 mg. per serving.

BRAND	ACCEPTABLE	NOT RECOMMENDED
	30% or less calories from fat 800 mg. sodium or less (LIMIT USE)	**Greater than 30% calories from fat greater than 800 mg. sodium**
Stouffer's Right Course (Cont'd)	▲*Chicken tenderloins in peanut sauce with linguini and vegetables* ▲Fiesta beef with corn pasta ▲Homestyle pot roast ▲*Sesame chicken* ▲*Shrimp primavera* ▲Sliced turkey in a mild curry sauce with rice pilaf ▲*Vegetarian chili*	

Swanson		Chicken pie
		Dinner:
		   Chopped sirloin beef
		   Fish 'n' chips
		   Fried chicken (dark portions)
		   Fried chicken (white portions)
		   Loin of pork
		   Meat loaf
		   Mexican style
		   Salisbury steak
		   Turkey (mostly white meat)
		Great Starts breakfast:
		   Belgian waffle and sausages
		   Belgian waffles and strawberries in sauce
		   French toast with sausages
		   Pancakes with sausages
		   Scrambled eggs and home fried potatoes

▲ High sodium, 400 mg. or greater per serving.

BRAND	ACCEPTABLE	NOT RECOMMENDED
	30% or less calories from fat 800 mg. sodium or less (LIMIT USE)	**Greater than 30% calories from fat greater than 800 mg. sodium**
Swanson (Cont'd)		Great Starts breakfast (Cont'd): 　Scrambled eggs and sausage with hashed 　　brown potatoes 　Scrambled eggs, home fried potatoes and 　　three bacon slices Homestyle Recipe Dinners: 　*Cheese ravioli* 　Chicken and noodles 　Chicken nibbles with french fried potatoes 　Deluxe chicken pie 　Fish 'n' chips 　Fried chicken and whipped potatoes 　*Lasagna with meat sauce* 　Macaroni and cheese 　Salisbury steak in gravy with macaroni 　　and cheese 　Scalloped potatoes and ham 　Sirloin tips in burgundy sauce with 　　noodles and vegetables in sauce 　Tuna noodle casserole 　Turkey in gravy with dressing and whipped 　　potatoes Hungry Man: 　Beef pot pie 　Chicken pot pie 　Meatloaf 　Turkey pot pie 　Yankee pot roast

Brand	**Acceptable**	**Not Recommended**
	30% or less calories from fat 800 mg. sodium or less (LIMIT USE)	Greater than 30% calories from fat greater than 800 mg. sodium
Swanson (Cont'd)		Hungry Man Dinners: Fried chicken (dark portions) Salisbury steak Turkey (mostly white meat) Original style: Beef pot pie Chicken pot pie Turkey pot pie
The Budget Gourmet	Budget Gourmet Light and Healthy Dinners: ▲Chicken breast parmigiana ▲Sirloin of beef in wine sauce ▲Stuffed turkey breast ▲Teriyaki chicken breast Slim Selects: ▲Glazed turkey ▲Mandarin chicken	Budget Gourmet Light: Beef stroganoff Linguini and scallops and chives Roast chicken and herb gravy Sirloin of beef in herb sauce Sliced turkey breast and herb gravy Budget Gourmet Light and Healthy Dinners: Beef pot roast Italian style meatloaf Sirloin salisbury steak Special recipe sirloin of beef Slim Selects: Cheese ravioli Chicken suiza enchiladas French recipe chicken and vegetables Ham and asparagus au gratin Lasagna with meat sauce Linguini with scallops and clams

▲ High sodium, 400 mg. or greater per serving.

BRAND	ACCEPTABLE	NOT RECOMMENDED
	30% or less calories from fat 800 mg. sodium or less (LIMIT USE)	**Greater than 30% calories from fat greater than 800 mg. sodium**

The Budget Gourmet
(Cont'd)
		Slim Selects (Cont'd):
		  Oriental beef
		  Sirloin of beef in herb sauce
		  Sirloin ranchero enchiladas
		  Sirloin salisbury steak

Tyson – Looney Tune Meals		Bugs Bunny chicken chunks Daffy Duck spaghetti and meat balls
Tyson Gourmet Selection	▲Chicken a l'orange ▲Chicken mesquite	Breast of turkey with dressing Chicken Francais Chicken marsala Chicken oriental Chicken picatta Chicken sweet and sour

Weight Watchers	▲Broccoli and cheese baked potato
	Fajitas:
	  ▲*Beef*
	  ▲Chicken
	▲*Fillet of fish au gratin*
	▲London broil in mushroom sauce
	▲Sweet 'n sour chicken tenders
		Baked cheese ravioli
		Beef salisbury steak romano
		Beef sirloin tips
		Beef stroganoff
		Breaded chicken cordon bleu
		Cheese manicotti
		Cheese pizza
		Chicken a la king
		Chicken burrito
		Chicken divan baked potato
		Chicken fettucini
		Chicken nuggets

▲ High sodium, 400 mg. or greater per serving.

BRAND	ACCEPTABLE	NOT RECOMMENDED
	30% or less calories from fat 800 mg. sodium or less (LIMIT USE)	Greater than 30% calories from fat greater than 800 mg. sodium

Weight Watchers (Cont'd)		*Chopped beef steak*
		Deluxe French bread pizza
		Enchiladas:
		  Beef ranchero
		  Cheese ranchero
		  Chicken suiza
		Garden lasagna
		Imperial chicken
		Italian cheese lasagna
		Lasagna with meat sauce
		Microwave breakfast:
		  English muffin sandwiches
		Oven fried fish
		Pasta primavera
		Pepperoni French bread pizza
		Sausage pizza
		Seafood linguini
		Southern fried chicken patty
		Spaghetti with meat sauce
		Stuffed sole with newburg sauce
		Stuffed turkey breast
		Veal patty parmigiana

Worthington		Vegetarian pie: *Chicken-like flavor*

Desserts

▨ No butterfat and/or added saturated fat (LIMIT USE)

Products listed in this category are preferred because they do not contain butterfat and/or other saturated fats. Some products, however, are high in total fat (e.g., regular Tofutti, Rice Dream, Ice Bean) and others are high in simple sugars. Therefore, limited consumption is recommended.

▨ Low Butterfat, 3 grams fat or less per serving (LIMIT USE)

Products listed in this category are generally made with low fat dairy products and are lower in saturated fat than most other frozen dairy desserts. Many of these products are also high in simple sugars. Limited intake is recommended.

NOT RECOMMENDED

▨ High butterfat, greater than 3 grams fat per serving, and/or contains other saturated fat

Products containing greater than 3 grams of butterfat per serving and/or other saturated fats are not recommended.

NOTE

■ The sodium content of frozen desserts in this section varies depending on type. Frozen juice or ice cream bars range from 5-110 mg. per 4 ounce serving. Frozen cake type desserts range from 200-350 mg. per 2½ ounce serving. Sodium symbols are used to indicate high (▲) or low (▽) sodium **only** when sodium content is provided on the product label. Those products that are not identified with either symbol may be either high or low sodium or contain between 141-399 mg. sodium per serving.

BRAND	ACCEPTABLE		NOT RECOMMENDED
	No butterfat and/or added saturated fat (LIMIT USE)	Low butterfat, 3 grams fat or less per serving (LIMIT USE)	High butterfat, greater than 3 grams fat per serving and/or contains other saturated fat
All brands	Fruit ice Sorbet	Sherbet	Ice cream Ice cream bars Ice cream sandwiches *Ice milk
Breyers		Lowfat frozen yogurt: ▽Strawberry ▽Vanilla Natural Light ice milk: ▽*Natural strawberry* ▽Vanilla raspberry parfait	Natural Light ice milk: *Chocolate* Chocolate fudge twirl Fudge toffee parfait Heavenly hash Natural vanilla Praline almond crunch Vanilla-chocolate-strawberry
Crystal Light	Crystal Light bars: ▽All flavors		Cool 'n Creamy bars: Chocolate amaretto *Chocolate-vanilla* Double chocolate fudge *Frozen bavarian* *Orange* *Vanilla*
Dannon			Frozen lowfat yogurt dipped in chocolate flavored coating: *Banana* *Raspberry* *Strawberry* *Vanilla*

▽ Low sodium, 140 mg. or less per serving.
* Certain lowfat varieties are available. See brand name listings.

BRAND	ACCEPTABLE		NOT RECOMMENDED
	No butterfat and/or added saturated fat (LIMIT USE)	Low butterfat, 3 grams fat or less per serving (LIMIT USE)	High butterfat, greater than 3 grams fat per serving and/or contains other saturated fat
DCA foods	3-D monster pops		
Disney Pops	Cherry Grape Orange		
Dole	Fresh Lites: ▽Pineapple-orange ▽*Raspberry* Fruit 'n Juice bars: ▽Peach passion fruit ▽Pineapple-orange-banana ▽Raspberry ▽Raspberry and pineapple orange ▽Strawberry Fruit sorbet: ▽*Mandarin* ▽*Raspberry* Sun Tops: ▽Real juice fruit bars	Fruit and yogurt: ▽Mixed berry ▽Strawberry-banana	
Dove			Light Bar: *Vanilla dipped in milk chocolate* Rondos bite size ice cream
Edy's Inspirations		▽•All natural frozen yogurt	Lowfat frozen yogurt: Cookies 'n cream

▽ Low sodium, 140 mg. or less per serving.
• Contains egg yolks.

BRAND	ACCEPTABLE		NOT RECOMMENDED
	No butterfat and/or added saturated fat (LIMIT USE)	Low butterfat, 3 grams fat or less per serving (LIMIT USE)	High butterfat, greater than 3 grams fat per serving and/or contains other saturated fat
Espirit		Soft frozen lowfat yogurt: ▽Peach ▽Strawberry ▽Vanilla	
Farm Foods	Ice bean: ▽†Carob super crunch ▽†Cherry vanilla ▽†Honey vanilla ▽†Strawberry		
Freezer Pleezer	▽Assorted pops Juice coolers: ▽Regular ▽Sugar free ▽Melon pops ▽Twin pops	▽Fudge bars ▽*Fudge cremes* ▽Orange creme treats ▽Sugar free fudge treats	*Delight bars* Ice milk bars Lite Bites: Raspberry
Haagen Dazs			Sorbet and cream: Blueberry and cream Key lime and cream Oranges and cream Raspberry and cream Special Editions: Deep chocolate peanut butter Macadamia brittle Vanilla and caramel triple nut

▽ Low sodium, 140 mg. or less per serving.
† High fat, limit use.

BRAND	ACCEPTABLE		NOT RECOMMENDED
	No butterfat and/or added saturated fat (LIMIT USE)	Low butterfat, 3 grams fat or less per serving (LIMIT USE)	High butterfat, greater than 3 grams fat per serving and/or contains other saturated fat
Jell-O	Citrus snowburst soft frozen drink bars: ▽Lemon ▽Orange Gelatin pops: ▽Variety pack		Pudding pops: Chocolate Chocolate lovers variety pack Chocolate-vanilla swirl Peanut butter-chocolate Vanilla
Kemps		Frozen yogurt: ▽Chocolate ▽Vanilla	
Klondike			Lite: Sugar free 97% fat free frozen dessert
Kool-Aid	Kool-Pops: ▽Merry berry pack ▽The punch bunch	▽Cream pops	
Kroger	Deluxe fat free: ▽Vanilla fudge swirl	Lite ice milk: ▽Chocolate ▽Vanilla ▽Vanilla, chocolate, strawberry Orange sherbet Sugar free deluxe: ▽Vanilla frozen dessert	Lite ice milk: Black forest Chocolate chip Cookies 'n cream Heavenly hash Vanilla Swiss almond
Lifesavers	▽Flavor pops		

▽ Low sodium, 140 mg. or less per serving.

BRAND	ACCEPTABLE		NOT RECOMMENDED
	No butterfat and/or added saturated fat (LIMIT USE)	Low butterfat, 3 grams fat or less per serving (LIMIT USE)	High butterfat, greater than 3 grams fat per serving and/or contains other saturated fat
Mars			3-Musketeers chocolate ice cream bar Snickers ice cream bar
Merritt Foods Company	Bomb Pop Jr.		
Micro Shake		Yogurt Micro Shake: ▽*Wildberry*	Yogurt Micro Shake: *Chocolate*
Rice Dream	Non-dairy dessert: ▽†*Carob* ▽†Lemon ▽†Strawberry ▽†Vanilla ▽†Wild berry		Non-dairy dessert: Carob chip Peanut butter fudge
Sara Lee			All butter pound cake Chocolate mousse Classic cheesecakes (4 individual) French cheesecake Strawberry French cheesecake
Savino	Sorbet: ▽All flavors		
Sealtest	Nonfat frozen yogurt: ▽Red raspberry ▽Vanilla ▽Vanilla, strawberry, chocolate		

▽ Low sodium, 140 mg. or less per serving.
† High fat, limit use.

BRAND	ACCEPTABLE		NOT RECOMMENDED
	No butterfat and/or added saturated fat (LIMIT USE)	Low butterfat, 3 grams fat or less per serving (LIMIT USE)	High butterfat, greater than 3 grams fat per serving and/or contains other saturated fat
Stroh's		Low-fat frozen yogurt: ▽Peach ▽Strawberry ▽Strawberry-banana	All natural new dairy dessert: Butter pecan Chocolate Heavenly hash Neapolitan Raspberry chocolate Vanilla
Texas Gold		Lite ice milk: ▽Chocolate ▽*Neapolitan* ▽Vanilla	Lite ice milk: *Cookies 'n cream* Heavenly hash
The Original Brand	Popsicle: ▽Ice pops ▽Sugar free ice pops	Creamsicle: ▽Sugar free cream pops Fudgsicle: ▽Sugar free fudge pops	Popsicle bars, sugar free: Vanilla flavored center, chocolate coating
Tofutti	Lite Lite Tofutti: Deep chocolate fudge ▽*Strawberry vanilla twirl* Regular Tofutti: ▽†Chocolate supreme ▽†Vanilla almond bark ▽†Wildberry supreme		Lite Lite Tofutti: Chocolate vanilla twirl Vanilla-chocolate-strawberry
Trix	▽Pops		

▽ Low sodium, 140 mg. or less per serving.
† High fat, limit use.

BRAND	ACCEPTABLE		NOT RECOMMENDED
	No butterfat and/or added saturated fat (LIMIT USE)	Low butterfat, 3 grams fat or less per serving (LIMIT USE)	High butterfat, greater than 3 grams fat per serving and/or contains other saturated fat
Weight Watchers	▽*Double fudge bars*	▽Chocolate treat Grand Collection premium ice milk: 　▽Neapolitan 　▽Vanilla ▽Sugar free orange vanilla treat Vanilla sandwich bars	*Boston cream pie* Cheesecake Chocolate brownie Chocolate cake German chocolate cake Raspberry mousse Strawberry cheesecake
Welch's	Fruit juice bars: 　▽Grape 　▽Raspberry 　▽Strawberry		
Yoplait		Soft frozen yogurt: 　▽*Raspberry* 　▽Raspberry vanilla swirl 　▽Strawberry 　▽Strawberry-banana swirl 　▽*Vanilla swirl*	

▽ Low sodium, 140 mg. or less per serving.

Vegetables

Frozen vegetables provide convenience in availability, storage and ease of preparation. They are excellent sources of vitamins and minerals but are often lower in fiber and higher in sodium than their fresh counterparts. Some frozen vegetables may also have added saturated fats.

ACCEPTABLE

■ **Without added fat or salt**

These are the preferred selections because they do not contain added fat or salt.

■ **May have added acceptable oil and/or salt**

These products are less desirable because they are higher in fat and/or sodium. Fried vegetables such as french fries or onion rings should be prepared without fat and consumed in limited amounts.

NOT RECOMMENDED

■ **With added saturated fat**

Frozen vegetable products that contain added saturated fat are not recommended.

NOTE

■ The average sodium content of frozen vegetables without added salt ranges between 15-40 mg. per $1/2$ cup serving. Vegetables frozen with added salt range between 100-200 mg. per $1/2$ cup serving. Frozen vegetables with added sauces or flavorings can contain between 350-600 mg. per $1/2$ cup serving. Sodium symbols are used to indicate high (▲) or low (▽) sodium **only** when sodium content is provided on the product label. Those products that are not identified with either symbol may be either high or low sodium or contain between 141-399 mg. sodium per serving.

BRAND	ACCEPTABLE		NOT RECOMMENDED
	Without added fat or salt	May have added acceptable oil and/or salt	With added saturated fat
Avondale			French fried potatoes French fried shoestring potatoes

Birds Eye	▽Broccoli cuts
	▽Broccoli spears
	▽Cooked winter squash
	▽Cut green beans
	Deluxe vegetables:
	  ▽★"Sugar snap" snap peas
	  ▽★Artichoke hearts
	  ▽*Baby cob corn*
	  ▽Whole baby carrots
	  ▽Whole green beans
	Farm Fresh mixtures:
	  ▽★Broccoli, baby carrots and water chestnuts
	  ▽★Broccoli, cauliflower and red peppers
	  ▽★Broccoli, cauliflower and carrots
	  ▽★Broccoli, corn and red peppers
	  ▽★Broccoli, green beans, pearl onions and red peppers
	  ▽Cauliflower, zucchini, carrots and red peppers
		Classics:
		  French green beans with toasted almonds
		  Italian style pasta salad
		  ▲*Pasta marinara*
		  ▲Peas and pearl onions
		Custom Cuisine:
		  ▲Vegetables with delicate herb sauce
		Deluxe vegetables:
		  ▽★Tender tiny peas
		French green beans with almonds
		▽★Green peas
		International Recipe:
		  ▲French style rice
		  New England style
		  ▲Stir-fry Chinese style
		  ▲Stir-fry Japanese style
		▽Mixed vegetables
		Salad:
		  †*Italian pasta*
		  ▲†*Three bean*
			Classics:
			  Broccoli with cheese sauce
			  Cauliflower with cheese sauce
			  Macaroni and cheese
			  Peas and potatoes with cream sauce
			  Potatoes au gratin
			Custom Cuisine:
			  Chow mein vegetables in oriental sauce
			  Pasta and vegetables in creamy stroganoff sauce
			  Vegetables with authentic oriental sauce
			  Vegetables with creamy mushroom sauce
			  Vegetables with dijon mustard sauce
			International Recipe:
			  Continental style pasta
			  Fettuccine alfredo
			  Japanese style
			  Scalloped potatoes florentine

▲ High sodium, 400 mg. or greater per serving.
▽ Low sodium, 140 mg. or less per serving.
† High fat, limit use.
★ High fiber, 3 g. or greater per serving.

BRAND	ACCEPTABLE		NOT RECOMMENDED
	Without added fat or salt	May have added acceptable oil and/or salt	With added saturated fat
Birds Eye (Cont'd)	Farm Fresh whole vegetables: ▽★Individual broccoli spears ▽Individual green beans ▽Individual whole green beans ▽★Italian green beans ▽Sweet corn		Salad: *Creamy pasta* *Creamy ranch* Tortellini
Budget Gourmet Side Dishes			Cauliflower in cheddar cheese sauce Cheddared potatoes Cheddared potatoes and broccoli Cheese tortellini *Glazed apples in raspberry sauce* Macaroni and cheese *Nacho potatoes* New England recipe vegetables *New potatoes in sour cream sauce* Oriental rice with vegetables Pasta alfredo with broccoli Peas and cauliflower in cream sauce *Peas and water chestnuts oriental* Rice pilaf with green beans Spinach au gratin Spring vegetables in cheese sauce Three-cheese potatoes Ziti in marinara sauce

▽ Low sodium, 140 mg. or less per serving.
★ High fiber, 3 g. or greater per serving.

BRAND	ACCEPTABLE		NOT RECOMMENDED
	Without added fat or salt	May have added acceptable oil and/or salt	With added saturated fat
Freshlike	▽Broccoli cut spears ▽California blend ▽•Capri: Vegetables with rotini pasta ▽Cut golden corn ▽Cut green beans ▽•Del Sol: Vegetables with shell pasta ▽Midwestern blend ▽Oriental blend ▽Sliced carrots	▽Green peas ▽Italian blend ▽Mixed vegetables	Micro Quick: Broccoli in cheese sauce Broccoli, pasta, carrots in cheese sauce Cauliflower in cheese sauce Corn in butter sauce Corn, Italian green beans, red peppers in butter sauce Peas in butter sauce Peas, carrots, onions in cheese sauce Peas, cauliflower, red peppers in butter sauce
Green Giant	Family size: Cut green beans ▽Niblets corn ▽Individually frozen broccoli spears ▽Niblet ears, 4 ears corn on the cob One serving: ▽Nibblers corn on the cob	Harvest Fresh: Cut broccoli Cut green beans ▽Niblets corn Sweet peas Rice Originals: ▲White 'n wild	Broccoli in cheese-flavored sauce Broccoli spears in butter sauce Broccoli, cauliflower and carrots in cheese flavored sauce Cauliflower in cheese flavored sauce Cut leaf spinach in butter sauce Garden Gourmet: Asparagus pilaf Creamy mushroom Fettuccine primavera *Pasta dijon* *Rotini cheddar* *Sherry wild rice*

▲ High sodium, 400 mg. or greater per serving.
▽ Low sodium, 140 mg. or less per serving.
• Contains egg yolks.

BRAND	ACCEPTABLE		NOT RECOMMENDED
	Without added fat or salt	May have added acceptable oil and/or salt	With added saturated fat
Green Giant (Cont'd)			LeSueur baby early peas in butter sauce
			Microwave:
			Broccoli cuts in butter sauce
			Broccoli in cheese flavored sauce
			Cauliflower in cheese flavored sauce
			Corn on the cob – two nibblers in butter sauce
			LeSueur baby early peas in butter sauce
			Niblets corn in butter sauce
			Niblets corn in butter sauce
			One serving:
			Baby peas in butter
			Cut broccoli in cheese
			Niblets corn in butter
			Pasta Accents:
			Creamy cheddar
			Garden herb seasoning
			Garlic seasoning
			Primavera
			Rice Originals:
			Medley
			Valley Combination:
			Broccoli-cauliflower medley
			Broccoli fanfare

BRAND	ACCEPTABLE		NOT RECOMMENDED
	Without added fat or salt	May have added acceptable oil and/or salt	With added saturated fat

Kroger	▽Asparagus spears
	▽Baby whole okra
	▽Blackeye peas
	▽Broccoli cuts
	▽Broccoli spears
	▽Brussels sprouts
	▽Cauliflower florets
	▽Chopped broccoli
	▽Chopped collard greens
	Chopped green peppers
	▽Chopped mustard greens
	▽Chopped onions
	▽Chopped spinach
	▽Chopped turnip greens
	▽Corn on the cob
	▽Corn tots
	▽Crinkle cut carrots
	▽Crowder peas
	▽Cut green beans
	▽Cut leaf spinach
	▽Cut okra
	▽French style green beans
	Garden Blend:
	  ▽Broccoli and cauliflower
	  ▽*California style vegetables*
	  ▽Oriental style vegetables
	  Vegetable gumbo mix
		▽Baby lima beans
		French Fried Potatoes:
		  ▽†Crinkle cut
		  †Regular
		  ▽†Shoestring
		  ▽†Steak fries
		Garden Blend:
		  ▽Italian style vegetables
		▽Green peas
		†Heat and eat taters
		▽Mixed vegetables
		†•Onion rings
		Pasta Plus:
		  ▽•*Bowtie salad*
		  ▽Seashell salad
		▽Peas and carrots
		†Tater rounds
		▽Vegetable soup mix
			French Fried Potatoes:
			  Potato wedges
			Just for one:
			  Cut broccoli spears in cheese sauce

▽ Low sodium, 140 mg. or less per serving.
• Contains egg yolks.
† High fat, limit use.

BRAND	ACCEPTABLE		NOT RECOMMENDED
	Without added fat or salt	May have added acceptable oil and/or salt	With added saturated fat
Kroger (Cont'd)	Just for one: ▽Cut broccoli spears ▽Cut whole kernel corn ▽Leaf spinach Pasta Plus: ▽Oriental salad ▽Rotini salad Shredded hash brown potatoes ▽Southern style hash brown potatoes ▽Speckled butter beans ▽Stew vegetables ▽Whole baby carrots ▽Whole kernel golden corn ▽Whole kernel golden sweet corn		
LaChoy	Snow peas		
McCains		▽†Crinkle cut golden superfries †Tasti taters golden superfries	
McKenzie's	Garden Fresh Mixtures: ▽Broccoli, cauliflower, carrots		
Micro Magic			Microwave: French fries Skinny fries Tater sticks

▽ Low sodium, 140 mg. or less per serving.
† High fat, limit use.

BRAND	ACCEPTABLE		NOT RECOMMENDED
	Without added fat or salt	**May have added acceptable oil and/or salt**	**With added saturated fat**
Moore's		•†Onion rings	
Mrs. Paul's		†Old fashioned onion rings	
Oh Boy			Stuffed Potatoes: With natural cheddar cheese With onion, sour cream and chives
Okray's	Hash brown potato patties		
Ore Ida	Chopped onions Hash Browns: Regular Southern style potatoes Potatoes O'Brien with onions and peppers	†Crispy crowns †Golden crinkles †Golden fries †Golden patties †Homestyle potato wedges with skins •Medley: Cauliflower, broccoli and carrots (with bread crumb coating) Microwave: †Crinkle cuts †Hash browns †Tater tots †•Mushrooms (with bread crumb coating) †Pixie crinkles †Shoestring french fried potatoes †Tater tots	Cheddar browns Crispers Lites: *Crinkle cuts* Onion ringers Toaster hash browns Twice baked cheese potato

• Contains egg yolks.
† High fat, limit use.

BRAND	ACCEPTABLE		NOT RECOMMENDED
	Without added fat or salt	**May have added acceptable oil and/or salt**	**With added saturated fat**
Ore Ida (Cont'd)		†Tater tots, seasoned with onions †•Zucchini (with bread crumb coating)	
Stokely's Singles	▽Baby whole carrots ▽Broccoli and cauliflower ▽*Broccoli, baby whole carrots and water chestnuts* ▽Broccoli, cauliflower and baby whole carrots ▽Cut broccoli spears ▽Cut corn ▽*Cut green beans* ▽*Mixed vegetables*	▲*Vegetables 'n rice in teriyaki sauce*	Broccoli, cauliflower and baby whole carrots in cheese sauce *Brussels sprouts in butter sauce* *Cauliflower in cheese sauce* *Corn on the cob in butter sauce* Cut broccoli spears in cheese sauce Shredded potatoes 'n vegetables in cheese sauce *Sweet peas in butter sauce* Vegetables 'n rotini in cheddar cheese sauce *Vegetables 'n shells in Italian style sauce*
Weight Watchers		Fancy Side Dishes: ▲*Oriental vegetables in an imperial sauce* ▲*Rice pilaf in seasoned sauce* *Whole baby carrots in a lemon glaze*	Fancy Side Dishes: *Cauliflower florets in a cheddar cheese sauce* *Fettucini alfredo with broccoli* *Pasta shells and cheese* *Potatoes au gratin in a zesty cheese sauce* *Vegetable medley in a cheddar cheese sauce*

▲ High sodium, 400 mg. or greater per serving.
▽ Low sodium, 140 mg. or less per serving.
• Contains egg yolks.
† High fat, limit use.

GRAIN PRODUCTS

This section contains listings with criteria for evaluating the following food categories:

◇ Bread
◇ Bread Crumbs, Croutons, Stuffing
◇ Cereals
◇ Pasta, Potato and Grain Mixes

Foods in these groups are rich sources of complex carbohydrates, B-vitamins, iron, zinc, magnesium and fiber. A greater variety of vitamins and minerals are found in whole grain products than in their refined or processed alternatives.

Whole grain products are also good sources of dietary fiber. When fiber information is provided on the label those foods containing 3 or more grams of fiber per serving are identified with the (★) fiber symbol. Remember that some fibers (i.e., water soluble fiber) found in oats, barley, legumes and pectin containing fresh fruits help to lower cholesterol levels and stabilize blood sugar levels. Therefore, these are especially good food choices.

Bread

■ Without added fat

Breads in this category are preferred because they contain no added fat.

■ With added unsaturated oil

These breads are acceptable choices. Although they contain fat, most have only 2 grams or less per slice.

With added acceptable partially hydrogenated oil or shortening

These breads contain added oils that have been hydrogenated to form shortening. These hydrogenated oils are acceptable as long as they are **not** from palm, palm kernel or coconut. Breads in this category are also low in fat, usually containing 2 grams fat or less per slice.

The fiber content of breads is usually not listed on the label. To ensure that you are getting a whole wheat bread product look for "whole wheat flour" or "ground whole wheat" listed as the **first** ingredient on the label. These breads may have other grain flours listed as subsequent ingredients but the major ingredient (i.e., first ingredient), should always be "whole".

Breads with whole grains listed as the first or major ingredient are identified with a (★) fiber symbol.

NOT RECOMMENDED

■ With added saturated fat

Breads with added saturated fats are not recommended.

NOTE

- Sodium content of breads and rolls varies between brands and can range between 85-250 mg. sodium per 1 ounce serving. Some breakfast breads may contain greater than 500 mg. sodium per serving. Sodium symbols are used to indicate high (▲) or low (▽) sodium **only** when sodium content is provided on the product label. Those products that are not identified with either symbol may be either high or low sodium or contain between 141-399 mg. sodium per serving.

BRAND	ACCEPTABLE			NOT RECOMMENDED
	Without added fat	With added unsaturated oil	With added acceptable partially hydrogenated oil or shortening	With added saturated fat
Armel's Original	Pocket pita: *Onion (6 pieces)* *White (6 pieces)* ▽*White (8 pieces)* ▽★*Whole wheat (8 pieces)*			
Aunt Millie's		▽Homestyle buttermilk bread Homestyle cracked wheat bread Homestyle oatmeal bread		
Awrey's Best	▽Oat bran bread		▽★100% Whole wheat Hotdog buns Oat bran hotdog buns *Oat bran sandwich buns* ▲Sandwich buns ▲Sesame sandwich buns ▽Wheat n' rye	Buttercrust: Multigrain bread White enriched bread
Beefsteak		Breads: Hearty rye: Seeded Hearty wheat *Onion rye*		

▲ High sodium, 400 mg. or greater per serving.
▽ Low sodium, 140 mg. or less per serving.
★ High fiber, 3 g. or greater per serving, and/or whole grain listed as first ingredient.

BRAND	ACCEPTABLE			NOT RECOMMENDED
	Without added fat	With added unsaturated oil	With added acceptable partially hydrogenated oil or shortening	With added saturated fat
Beefsteak (Cont'd)		Breads (Cont'd): ▽Robust white Soft rye: No seeds Soft wheat bread		
Brownberry			▽*Apple honey wheat bread* Bakery Light: ▽Golden wheat ▽Italian ▽Oatmeal ▽Soft rye Bran'nola: ★Country oat ★Hearty wheat ▽★Nutty grain ★Original Natural dill rye bread ★Natural health nut bread ▽Natural oatmeal bread Natural pumpernickel rye bread Natural sandwich dark bread ▽Natural sandwich oatmeal	

▽ Low sodium, 140 mg. or less per serving.
★ High fiber, 3 g. or greater per serving, and/or whole grain listed as first ingredient.

BRAND	ACCEPTABLE			NOT RECOMMENDED
	Without added fat	With added unsaturated oil	With added acceptable partially hydrogenated oil or shortening	With added saturated fat
Brownberry (Cont'd)			★Natural wheat bread ▽Natural white bread Natural whole bran bread ▽Oatmeal raisin ▽*Orange raisin bread* ▽Raisin cinnamon bread ▽Raisin walnut bread ▽Sandwich oatmeal ▽Sandwich white bread ▽Soft wheat bread	
Chicago Hearth		Onion rolls Sour dough bread: 　San Francisco style	Heidelberg dill rye Jewish pumpernickel Sour dough bread: 　French bread	
Cole's				Homestyle garlic loaf: 　Oatbran 　Regular 　Romano cheese 　Seasoned Homestyle onion loaf
Country Oven			White enriched bread	
Country Oven Hearth		★100% stone ground 　whole wheat Deli rye Indian grain bread		6 Onion rolls Brown-n-serve: 　Bakers dozen hard rolls Cinnamon loaf

▽ Low sodium, 140 mg. or less per serving.
★ High fiber, 3 g. or greater per serving, and/or whole grain listed as first ingredient.

BRAND	ACCEPTABLE			NOT RECOMMENDED
	Without added fat	With added unsaturated oil	With added acceptable partially hydrogenated oil or shortening	With added saturated fat

Country Oven Hearth (Cont'd)		▽Light rice bran and barley
		▽Light wheat
				Kaiser rolls:
				  12 Gourmet enriched
				  6 Extra-large
				Rye bread:
				  American
				  Dark Jewish
				  Dark pumpernickel
				  Dill
				  Light Jewish
				  Olde Chicago
				  Warsaw pumpernickel
				San Francisco style sour French bread
				Sourdough enriched bread
				Split top wheat with oatbran bread
				Thin cocktail rye bread

Cybros	▽★*Low sodium whole wheat* ★Seven grain			
Food For Life		Wheat free: White rye bread Wheat free gluten free rice bread		

▽ Low sodium, 140 mg. or less per serving.
★ High fiber, 3 g. or greater per serving, and/or whole grain listed as first ingredient.

BRAND	ACCEPTABLE			NOT RECOMMENDED
	Without added fat	With added unsaturated oil	With added acceptable partially hydrogenated oil or shortening	With added saturated fat
Frankenmuth Valley				Cinnamon bread Fruit bread stollen Raisin bread Sourdough bread White bread
Holsum		▽King size white enriched bread		
Home Pride				Buttertop: Light wheat Light white Wheat White Wheat bread *White bread*
Kangaroo	Pocket bread: Onion White ★Whole wheat			
King's				Hawaiian bread Hawaiian rolls
Koepplinger's	Jewish pumpernickel No sugar Jewish rye bread *Raisin bran bread*	•*Jewish egg bread* •Jewish kaiser rolls •Jewish onion rolls Sliced French bread	Black Russian bread ▽Bohemian style bread Dinner rolls: ▽•White	Buttersweet: Wheat bread White bread Buttery cinnamon raisin bread

▽ Low sodium, 140 mg. or less per serving.
★ High fiber, 3 g. or greater per serving, and/or whole grain listed as first ingredient.
• Contains egg yolks.

BRAND	ACCEPTABLE			NOT RECOMMENDED
	Without added fat	With added unsaturated oil	With added acceptable partially hydrogenated oil or shortening	With added saturated fat

Koepplinger's (Cont'd)	Raisin bread
	Soft sticks
	Staff o' Life health bread:
	  ▽Oat bran
	  ▽Regular
	  ▽*Rice bran*
	  ▽Wheat bran
			▽Early American white bread
			Natural rye:
			  Caraway seeds
			  Seedless
			★Natural wheat bread
			Staff o' Life health bread:
			  Oatbran hot dog buns
				Hamburger buns:
				  Wheat
				  White
				Hot dog buns:
				  Wheat
				  White
				Italian bread sticks
				Perfect Harvest:
				  Wheat
				  White
				Submarine rolls

Kroger	Lite:
	  •Wheat
	  •White
	★Lite sandwich buns
		Brown-n-Serve:
		  Combo pack
		  Flake rolls
		  French stix
		  Italian stix
		  Krusty rolls:
		    Enriched with oat bran
		  Twin rolls
		Buttermilk:
		  ▽Sandwich enriched bread
			★100% whole wheat bread
			Black Forest rye bread
			▲Cottage rye
			Low sodium:
			  ▽Wheat
			  ▽White
			Multigrain bread
			Premium raisin bread
			Raisin bread
			Rye
			Wheat bread
				Buttercrust:
				  Lite multigrain
				  Lite wheat
				  Multigrain
				  Wheat
				  White
				Cracked wheat bread
				Deli style hoagie rolls
				Texas toast:
				  Enriched bread

▲ High sodium, 400 mg. or greater per serving.
▽ Low sodium, 140 mg. or less per serving.
★ High fiber, 3 g. or greater per serving, and/or whole grain listed as first ingredient.
• Contains egg yolks.

BRAND	ACCEPTABLE			NOT RECOMMENDED
	Without added fat	With added unsaturated oil	With added acceptable partially hydrogenated oil or shortening	With added saturated fat
Kroger (Cont'd)		▽Buttermilk sandwich bread Hot dog enriched buns Jumbo enriched buns ★Oat bran buns Sandwich enriched buns Sesame enriched buns Sesame seeded Italian style bread Wheat hot dog buns Wheat sandwich buns White enriched bread		
Marshalls	★Spring wheat bread	★•Dinner rolls ★•Hamburger buns ★•Hot dog buns		7-grain bread
Marty Bread		13 grains and seeds		

Natural Grains		Corn bran bread
		Honey wheat bread
		▽Lite oat bran bread
		Rice bran bread
			★12 Grains
			Hi-fiber bread
			Lite:
			  ▽Multigrain
			  ▽Wheat
			  ▽White
			★Oat bran bread
			Oatmeal bread
			★Stone ground whole wheat
				7 whole grains bread
				European rye bread

▽ Low sodium, 140 mg. or less per serving.
★ High fiber, 3 g. or greater per serving, and/or whole grain listed as first ingredient.
• Contains egg yolks.

BRAND	ACCEPTABLE			NOT RECOMMENDED
	Without added fat	With added unsaturated oil	With added acceptable partially hydrogenated oil or shortening	With added saturated fat
Nature's Orchard				Apple bread Cherry nut bread
Oatmeal Goodness		▽*Cinnamon oatmeal bread* ▽Oatmeal and bran bread ▽Oatmeal and sunflower seeds ▽Wheat oatmeal bread ▽*White oatmeal bread, thinner sliced*	Light: ▽Bran and oat	

Pastry Shoppe	Crusty French bagguette
	Crusty lecharm boule
	Lite breads:
	  ★Wheat
	  White
	Lite multigrain bread
		•Bran knot rolls
		Caraway rye rolls
		•Cinnamon loaf
		Cocktail rye party bread
		▽Corn bran bread
		Crusty dill rye loaf
		Crusty pumpernickel raisin loaf
		Crusty rye onion rolls
		Crusty rye/sauerkraut loaf
		•*Egg demi loaf*
		•Egg kaiser rolls
		English toasting bread
			Dinner rolls:
			  Enriched
			  ★*Oat bran*
			Garlic bread
			Light caraway rye bread
			Light rye rolls
			Round rye/onion loaf
			★*Wheat/Italian bread*
				Garden bread with cheese
				Garlic sticks

▽ Low sodium, 140 mg. or less per serving.
★ High fiber, 3 g. or greater per serving, and/or whole grain listed as first ingredient.
• Contains egg yolks.

BRAND	ACCEPTABLE			NOT RECOMMENDED
	Without added fat	With added unsaturated oil	With added acceptable partially hydrogenated oil or shortening	With added saturated fat

Pastry Shoppe (Cont'd)		English toasting rolls
		•Enriched egg bread
		French bread
		Hard rolls
		Hoagie rolls
		Hot dog buns:
		   Plain
		Italian style bread
		•Kaiser rolls
		Knot rolls:
		   •Bran
		   •Egg
		Natural grain bread
		Natural grain rolls
		Oat bran bread
		Oat bran rolls
		•Onion rolls
		Pumpernickel rolls
		Pumpernickel rye bread
		Raisin bread
		▽Rice bran bread
		Round light Jewish
		   rye bread
		▽Salt free white bread
		Sandwich buns:
		   Plain		

▽ Low sodium, 140 mg. or less per serving.
• Contains egg yolks

BRAND	ACCEPTABLE			NOT RECOMMENDED
	Without added fat	With added unsaturated oil	With added acceptable partially hydrogenated oil or shortening	With added saturated fat
Pastry Shoppe (Cont'd)		Snowflake rolls Sour dough rolls Submarine rolls Wheat bread Wheat buns Wheat rolls White bread *White party bread*		

Pepperidge Farm			▽Cinnamon bread
			Classic dark
			  pumpernickel bread
			Club rolls
			▽Cracked wheat bread
			Distinctive white bread:
			  Toasting
			Family rye bread:
			  Seeded
			  Seedless
			Frankfurter rolls
			French bread (loaf)
			French rolls:
			  ▲2-rolls
			  4-rolls
			  9-rolls
			  Brown and serve
			    3-rolls
			Hamburger rolls
				Butter crescents
				Dinner rolls
				Distinctive white bread:
				  Family
				  Original
				  Sandwich
				Golden twists
				Oatmeal bread:
				  Regular
				  Thin sliced
				Original white bread
				Party rolls
				Stone ground 100% whole
				  wheat bread

▲ High sodium, 400 mg. or greater per serving.
▽ Low sodium, 140 mg. or less per serving.

BRAND	ACCEPTABLE			NOT RECOMMENDED
	Without added fat	With added unsaturated oil	With added acceptable partially hydrogenated oil or shortening	With added saturated fat

Pepperidge Farm (Cont'd)			▽Hearth rolls
			Hearty slices:
			   Country white
			   ★Crunchy oat
			   ★Sesame wheat
			Light style:
			   ▽Oatmeal
			   ▽Vienna
			Onion sandwich buns
			Party rye bread
			Raisin bread
			▽Raisin with cinammon
			Sandwich buns
			Sourdough rolls:
			  9-rolls
			Thin sliced dijon rye,
			  seedless bread
			Very Thin:
			  Oatmeal
			  ▽★Wheat
			  ▽White
			▽Vienna bread
			Wheat bread	

Pritikin	▽★Rye bread ▽★Stone ground whole wheat			

▽ Low sodium, 140 mg. or less per serving.
★ High fiber, 3 g. or greater per serving, and/or whole grain listed as first ingredient.

BRAND	ACCEPTABLE			NOT RECOMMENDED
	Without added fat	With added unsaturated oil	With added acceptable partially hydrogenated oil or shortening	With added saturated fat
Roman Meal		Honey and oat bran Roman Light: ▽Seven grain ▽Wheat	Roman Light: ▽Oat bran n' honey	
Rosen's	Jewish pumpernickel Reduced calorie: ▽Jewish caraway rye ▽Jewish pumpernickel	•Egg bread •French bread		
Rubschlager	▽★Danish pumpernickel bread	▽Cocktail rye bread Jewish rye bread		
Safari	Pita bread: ★100% whole wheat, large ★100% whole wheat, small White			
Schafer's		Country Hearth: Deli rye *Honey nut 'n oat bran* Indian grain ▽*Oat bran* Italian bread	▽Hillbilly old fashioned bread	

▽ Low sodium, 140 mg. or less per serving.
★ High fiber, 3 g. or greater per serving, and/or whole grain listed as first ingredient.
• Contains egg yolks.

BRAND	ACCEPTABLE			NOT RECOMMENDED
	Without added fat	With added unsaturated oil	With added acceptable partially hydrogenated oil or shortening	With added saturated fat
Schafer's (Cont'd)		Less: ▽Light Dark n' grainy ▽Lite oat bran ▽Lite wheat ★Lite wheat buns Lite white		
Sun Gold				White enriched bread
Taystee		▽D'Italiano real Italian bread Eights enriched buns	▽Giant enriched bread	Golden split top: Enriched Wheat
Toufayan's			Snuggles – hot dog buns	
Wonder	Light: ▽★Italian ▽Oatmeal ▽Wheat ▽White	Enriched Bread: ▽Big ▽Giant ▽Small Family Italian bread Light: ★Hamburger buns ★Hotdog buns ▽★Soft 100% wholewheat bread		

▽ Low sodium, 140 mg. or less per serving.
★ High fiber, 3 g. or greater per serving, and/or whole grain listed as first ingredient.

BRAND	ACCEPTABLE			NOT RECOMMENDED
	Without added fat	With added unsaturated oil	With added acceptable partially hydrogenated oil or shortening	With added saturated fat
BREAKFAST BREADS:				
All brands				*Coffee cakes *Croissants *Doughnuts *Pastries *Sweet rolls
Aldons			Oat bran English muffins	

Aunt Jemima			French toast:
			  ▲•*Cinnamon*
			  •Original
			▲•Frozen pancake batter
			Microwave pancakes:
			  ▲•Blueberry
			  ▲•Buttermilk
			  ▲•★Lite buttermilk
			  ▲•Original
			Waffles:
			  •Apple and cinnamon
			  •Blueberry
			  •Buttermilk
			  •Original
			  Whole grain and oat
			    bran
				French toast:
				  Original extra thick slices

▲ High sodium, 400 mg. or greater per serving.
★ High fiber, 3 g. or greater per serving, and/or whole grain listed as first ingredient.
• Contains egg yolks.
* These products may contain acceptable fats but are not recommended because they are high in total fat and/or simple sugar.

BRAND	ACCEPTABLE			NOT RECOMMENDED
	Without added fat	With added unsaturated oil	With added acceptable partially hydrogenated oil or shortening	With added saturated fat
Awrey's Best	Lowfat cholesterol free muffins: ▲Country bran		Lowfat cholesterol free muffins: ▲Country blueberry Muffins: •Banana pecan •Blueberry •Home style bran Oatbran *Pineapple raisin oatbran*	
Bays				English muffins
Belgian Chef			★Frozen waffles	
Dairy Fresh			English muffins: ★Oat bran	English muffins: Plain Raisin cinnamon
Downeyflake			Waffles: ▲•Blueberry ▲•Buttermilk ▲•Jumbo size ▲•★Multi-grain	
Entenmann's			Muffins: •Blueberry	Fruit and Fibre muffins: Honey raisin bran Muffins: *Oat bran*

▲ High sodium, 400 mg. or greater per serving.
★ High fiber, 3 g. or greater per serving, and/or whole grain listed as first ingredient.
• Contains egg yolks.

BRAND	ACCEPTABLE			NOT RECOMMENDED
	Without added fat	With added unsaturated oil	With added acceptable partially hydrogenated oil or shortening	With added saturated fat
Forcrest Foods, Ltd.	*Canadian style crumpets*			

Health Valley		Oat bran fancy fruit muffins:
		  ▽★*Almonds and dates*
		  ▽★*Blueberry*
		  ▽★*Raisin*		

Hostess		Mini muffins:
		  •Banana walnut
		  •Blueberry
		  •Cinnamon apple
		Oat bran muffins		

Howard Johnson			Toastees:
			  •Corn toaster muffins
				Toastees:
				  Blueberry toaster muffins

International	Bagels:
	  Blueberry
	  ▽*Cinnamon raisin*
	  •*Egg*
	  Oat bran
	  Onion
	  Plain			

Keebler			Elfin loaves:
			  Banana
			  •*Blueberry*	

▽ Low sodium, 140 mg. or less per serving.
★ High fiber, 3 g. or greater per serving, and/or whole grain listed as first ingredient.
• Contains egg yolks.

BRAND	ACCEPTABLE			NOT RECOMMENDED
	Without added fat	With added unsaturated oil	With added acceptable partially hydrogenated oil or shortening	With added saturated fat
Kellogg's			Eggo waffles: •Blueberry •Buttermilk Common Sense oat bran Common Sense oat bran with fruit and nuts ★Corn, wheat, rice and oat bran Nutri Grain •Homestyle •Nut and Honey Nutri Grain Raisin and Bran Nutri Grain •Strawberry Pop-tarts: Blueberry Brown sugar cinnamon Strawberry	
Kroger	Bagels: *Blueberry* •Egg ▽Onion	Bagels: Cinnamon raisin *Raisin 'n honey*	English muffins (in cardboard trays, refrigerator section): Plain	

▽ Low sodium, 140 mg. or less per serving.
★ High fiber, 3 g. or greater per serving, and/or whole grain listed as first ingredient.
• Contains egg yolks.

BRAND	ACCEPTABLE			NOT RECOMMENDED
	Without added fat	**With added unsaturated oil**	**With added acceptable partially hydrogenated oil or shortening**	**With added saturated fat**
Kroger (Cont'd)	Bagels (Cont'd): Plain *Wheat 'n honey*	English muffins (in cardboard trays, bread section): Oat bran Plain Raisin Sourdough ★Wheat Muffins: ★Corn bran	▲English muffins (in red canister, refrigerator section) ▲•Frozen pre-baked waffles ▲•Microwave buttermilk pancakes Muffins: Apple spice Banana nut Blueberry ★Multigrain Toaster Treats: ▽Strawberry	
Lenders	Bagelettes: Plain Bagels: Blueberry •Egg Garlic ★Oat bran Onion Plain	Bagelettes: ▽Cinnamon raisin Bagels: Cinnamon raisin		
Motor City Muffins		Muffin/Loaf: •Zucchini nut	Muffin/Loaf: •Apple-cinnamon-oatmeal	Muffin/Loaf: Banana chocolate chip Chocolate chip

▲ High sodium, 400 mg. or greater per serving.
▽ Low sodium, 140 mg. or less per serving.
★ High fiber, 3 g. or greater per serving, and/or whole grain listed as first ingredient.
• Contains egg yolks.

BRAND	ACCEPTABLE			NOT RECOMMENDED
	Without added fat	**With added unsaturated oil**	**With added acceptable partially hydrogenated oil or shortening**	**With added saturated fat**
Motor City Muffins (Cont'd)		Muffin/Loaf (eggless) (Cont'd): ★Blueberry nut oatbran ★Carrot cake oat bran ★Cherry oat bran ★Cranberry nut oat bran ★Cranberry oat bran ★Date oat bran ★Fig oat bran ★Peach oat bran ★Pineapple oat bran ★Raisin oat bran ★Strawberry oat bran ★Wild berry oat bran	Muffin/Loaf (Cont'd): •Banana nut •Blueberry •Blueberry oatbran •Blueberry oatmeal •Peanut butter chip •Pineapple (sugarless) •Poppyseed •Pumpkin •Whole wheat banana	
Nature's Warehouse		Pastry poppers: ▽Apple ▽Cherry ▽Raspberry ▽Strawberry		
Oatmeal Goodness		English muffins: *Cinnamon raisin oatmeal* *Honey oatmeal*		

▽ Low sodium, 140 mg. or less per serving.
★ High fiber, 3 g. or greater per serving, and/or whole grain listed as first ingredient.
• Contains egg yolks.

BRAND	ACCEPTABLE			NOT RECOMMENDED
	Without added fat	With added unsaturated oil	With added acceptable partially hydrogenated oil or shortening	With added saturated fat
Our very own	English muffins: *Cinnamon raisin* *Plain*			
Pastry Shoppe	Bagels: Blueberry •Egg Garlic Onion •Plain Wheat and honey	Bagels: *Pumpernickel* Raisin 'n honey Mini muffins: •Banana nut Oatbran, raisin and blueberry •Raisin bran Muffins: •Bran •Honey bran •Oat bran •Raisin honey bran •Raspberry honey bran	Muffins: •Almond poppy creme cake •Banana nut •Blueberry •Fruit	Muffins: Chocolate chip Strawberry cream cheese
Pepperidge Farm			English muffins: Cinnamon apple Cinnamon raisin Muffins: •Blueberry •Corn	English muffins: *Cinnamon chip* Plain

• Contains egg yolks.

BRAND	ACCEPTABLE			NOT RECOMMENDED
	Without added fat	With added unsaturated oil	With added acceptable partially hydrogenated oil or shortening	With added saturated fat
Pritikin	▽★English muffins			
Sara Lee	Bagels: 　Cinnamon and raisin 　Oat bran 　▲Onion 　▲Plain 　▲Poppy seed		Hearty fruit muffins: 　★Blueberry 　▲★Raisin bran 　★Oat bran muffins	
Sun Maid				Raisin English muffins
Thomas		English muffins: 　★Oat bran	English muffins: 　★Honey wheat 　Plain 　Raisin 　Sourdough	
TLC	Buttermilk crumpet Canadian style crumpet			*Cheese crumpets*
Weight Watchers	Microwave breakfast: 　•French toast with 　　cinnamon		Microwave breakfast: 　•Buttermilk pancakes 　▲•Pancakes with 　　blueberry topping	
Wonder		English muffins: 　Plain 　Raisin rounds		

▲ High sodium, 400 mg. or greater per serving.
▽ Low sodium, 140 mg. or less per serving.
★ High fiber, 3 g. or greater per serving, and/or whole grain listed as first ingredient.
• Contains egg yolks.

BRAND	ACCEPTABLE			NOT RECOMMENDED
	Without added fat	With added unsaturated oil	With added acceptable partially hydrogenated oil or shortening	With added saturated fat
REFRIGERATED AND FROZEN DOUGHS:				
Aldons			Frozen bread dough: 　Enriched white 　Oat bran 　Stone ground honey 　　wheat 　White dinner rolls	
Kroger		Frozen bread dough: 　White	▲French style croissants Oat bran breadsticks Texas style biscuits: 　▲Butter flavor 　▲Buttermilk 　▲Homestyle	Biscuits: 　Big flaky buttermilk 　Butter-me-not 　Buttermilk 　Homestyle Crescent dinner rolls Hot 'n Fresh: 　Soft breadsticks 　*White*
Merico			Hot 'n fresh soft 　breadsticks	*French style croissants*
Pastry Shoppe				Croissants: 　All butter 　Honey wheat
Pillsbury			Biscuits: 　Buttermilk 　Country	10 Tender layer biscuits: 　Buttermilk All ready pizza crust

▲ High sodium, 400 mg. or greater per serving.

Brand	Acceptable			Not Recommended
	Without added fat	With added unsaturated oil	With added acceptable partially hydrogenated oil or shortening	With added saturated fat

Pillsbury (Cont'd)			▽Crusty French loaf
			Heat 'n Eat:
			  ▲Biscuits
				Big Country biscuits:
				  Butter tastin'
				  Buttermilk
				Biscuits:
				  1869 Brand Buttermilk
				Cornbread twists
				Crescent dinner rolls
				Fillable pastry pocket
				Hungry Jack:
				  Butter tastin' flaky biscuits
				  Buttermilk flaky
				  Flaky biscuits
				  Honey flaky biscuits
				Pipin' Hot loaf:
				  Wheat
				  White
				Soft breadsticks

Rich's			Frozen bread dough: Enriched white	
Roman Meal			▲Biscuits Breadsticks	

▲ High sodium, 400 mg. or greater per serving.
▽ Low sodium, 140 mg. or less per serving.

Bread Crumbs, Croutons, Stuffing

ACCEPTABLE

■ **Without added fat**
These items are preferred because they have no added fat.

■ **With added unsaturated oil (LIMIT USE),** and

■ **With added acceptable partially hydrogenated oil or shortening (LIMIT USE)**
Products in these two latter categories are acceptable. Some products are higher in fat and sodium than others. Limited use is suggested.

NOT RECOMMENDED

■ **With added saturated fat**
Products with added saturated fat are not recommended.

NOTE

■ The sodium content of these foods is variable ranging from 95 mg. to 690 mg. sodium per 1 ounce serving. Sodium symbols are used to indicate high (▲) or low (▽) sodium **only** when sodium content is provided on the product label. Those products that are not identified with either symbol may be either high or low sodium or contain between 141-399 mg. sodium per serving.

BRAND	ACCEPTABLE			NOT RECOMMENDED
	Without added fat	With added unsaturated oil (LIMIT USE)	With added acceptable partially hydrogenated oil or shortening (LIMIT USE)	With added saturated fat
Betty Crocker				Stuffing mix: *Chicken flavor*
Bookbinders				Bread crumbs: Fish and seafood
Brownberry			Croutons: Caesar salad Onion and garlic Seasoned *Sage and onion stuffing*	Croutons: Cheddar cheese Cheese and garlic
Country Oven				Bread crumbs: Cheese seasoned – Italian style Unseasoned – American style
Devonsheer			Croutons: ▽*Onion and garlic* ▽Plain ▽*Seasoned*	Croutons: *Cheese and garlic*
Jason			Bread crumbs: *Flavored* *Plain*	
Kellogg's	Corn flake crumbs		Croutettes: Stuffing mix	

▽ Low sodium, 140 mg. or less per serving.

BRAND	ACCEPTABLE			NOT RECOMMENDED
	Without added fat	With added unsaturated oil (LIMIT USE)	With added acceptable partially hydrogenated oil or shortening (LIMIT USE)	With added saturated fat

Koepplinger's				Bread crumbs:
				  Regular
				  Seasoned
				Stuffing mixes:
				  Herb
				  Sage and onion
				  Seasoned crouton

Kroger			Croutons:
			  ▽Oat bran
			  Onion garlic
			  Seasoned
			  ▽Toasted
				Croutons:
				  Cheddar cheese
				Stuffing Magic:
				  Chicken flavor
				  Cornbread
				  Pork

Lawry's			Salad nuggets:
			  Onion
			  Plain
				Salad nuggets:
				  Garlic cheese

Nabisco	▽Cracker meal			

Old London				Bread crumbs:
				  Italian
				  Regular

Pepperidge Farm			Croutons:
			  Onion and garlic
			  Seasoned
				Croutons:
				  Cheddar and romano
				  cheese

▽ Low sodium, 140 mg. or less per serving.

BRAND	ACCEPTABLE			NOT RECOMMENDED
	Without added fat	**With added unsaturated oil (LIMIT USE)**	**With added acceptable partially hydrogenated oil or shortening (LIMIT USE)**	**With added saturated fat**

Pepperidge Farm (Cont'd)			Distinctive Stuffing:
			   Apple and raisin
			 Stuffing mixes:
			   Corn bread
			   ▲Cubed country style
			   ▲Cubed herb seasoned
			   ▲Herb seasoned
				Croutons (Cont'd):
				   Sour cream and chive
				 Distinctive Stuffing:
				   Classic chicken
				   Country garden herb
				   Harvest vegetable and almond
				   Wild rice and mushroom

Progresso				Italian bread crumbs

Reese			Croutons:
			   ▲Caesar salad
			   Onion and garlic
				Croutons:
				   Cheddar
				   Seasoned
				   Toasted

Salad Crispins				American style Homestyle Italian style

Stove Top				Microwave stuffing mix:
				   Broccoli and cheese
				   Chicken flavor
				   Homestyle corn bread
				 Stuffing mixes:
				   Chicken flavor
				   Cornbread
				   Homestyle herb
				   Long grain and wild rice
				   Pork

▲ High sodium, 400 mg. or greater per serving.

Cereals

ACCEPTABLE

■ **High fiber (3 grams or greater), no added fat**
These cereals are preferred choices because of their high fiber, low fat content. Some cereals may contain small amounts of nuts.

■ **High fiber (3 grams or greater), contains acceptable oil (may be partially hydrogenated)**
These cereals are high in dietary fiber but contain greater amounts of fat.

■ **Low fiber or fiber content unknown, may contain acceptable oil (may be partially hydrogenated)**
These cereals are acceptable but are low in dietary fiber and may contain added fat.

NOT RECOMMENDED

■ **With added saturated fat**
Cereals that contain added saturated fat are not recommended.

NOTE

■ Some cereals are high in simple sugar, such as added sucrose, honey, brown sugar, corn syrup and/or other sweeteners, fruit or fruit juice. There is scientific evidence to support that dietary sugar contributes to the development of dental caries. The *Dietary Guidelines for Americans, 3RD edition*[45] recommends that foods high in sugar be consumed in moderation by most healthy people and sparingly by people who need to limit their calorie intake. Because the sugar content of many cereals was unavailable at the time of publication, we were unable to categorize cereals based on sugar content. Individuals with high triglycerides, obesity, diabetes or reactive hypoglycemia are encouraged to limit their intake of simple sugar.

■ The sodium content of cereal can vary greatly depending on the processing. For example, regular oatmeal contains 0 mg. sodium. On the other hand, some instant oatmeals contain 200 mg. sodium per 1 ounce serving. Sodium symbols are used to indicate high (▲) or low (▽) sodium **only** when sodium content is provided on the product label. Those products that are not identified with either symbol may be either high or low sodium or contain between 141-399 mg. sodium per serving.

BRAND	ACCEPTABLE			NOT RECOMMENDED
	High fiber (3 grams or greater) no added fat	High fiber (3 grams or greater) contains acceptable oil (may be partially hydrogenated)	Low fiber or fiber content unknown, may contain acceptable oil (may be partially hydrogenated)	With added saturated fat
Alpen			Muesli with raisins and nuts: ▽No sugar or salt added	Muesli with raisins and nuts: Plain
American Home Foods	▽★Wheatena		▽Maypo oatmeal	
Arrowhead Mills	▽★*Nature O's* ▽★Oat bran ▽★*Raw wheat germ* ▽★*Wheat bran* (12 grams fiber)		▽Rice and Shine	
Barbara's	▽★*High fiber breakfast biscuits*	100% Crunchy oat bran: ▽★Blueberry ▽★Raisin ▽★Regular	Breakfast O's Corn flakes	
Breadshop	▽★Oat bran ▽★Triple bran	Nectar-Sweet granola: ▽★Crunchy oat bran ▽★Raspberry 'n Cream		Nectar-Sweet granola: Blueberry 'n Cream
Cost Cutter	★Raisin bran		Corn flakes Crispy rice	
El Molino			▽Puffed corn ▽Puffed rice ▽Puffed wheat	

▽ Low sodium, 140 mg. or less per serving.
★ High fiber, 3 g. or greater per serving.

BRAND	ACCEPTABLE			NOT RECOMMENDED
	High fiber (3 grams or greater) no added fat	**High fiber (3 grams or greater) contains acceptable oil (may be partially hydrogenated)**	**Low fiber or fiber content unknown, may contain acceptable oil (may be partially hydrogenated)**	**With added saturated fat**
Erewhon	▽★Fruit n' Wheat ▽★Raisin bran ▽★Super-O's ▽★Wheat flakes		Instant oatmeal: 　▽Apple cinnamon 　Apple raisin 　▽Maple spice	
Familia	Mixed cereal with fruit and nuts: 　▽★*25% Bran*		▽Crunchy Swiss Muesli Genuine Swiss Muesli: 　▽Original Mixed cereal with fruit and nuts: 　▽No added sugar 　▽Original recipe ▽Swiss baby cereal: 　No added sugar	
General Mills	Clusters: 　▽★Almonds, walnuts, pecans 　▽★Fiber One (13 grams fiber) Total oatmeal: 　▽★Apple cinnamon 　▽★*Cinnamon, raisin, almond* 　★Regular 　★Total raisin bran	▽★Raisin Nut Bran	Apple Cinnamon Cheerios Basic 4 Cheerios Cinnamon Toast Crunch Cocoa Puffs Count Chocula ▽Crispy Wheats 'n Raisins Golden Grahams Honey Nut Cheerios	*Fruity Yummy Mummy*

▽ Low sodium, 140 mg. or less per serving.
★ High fiber, 3 g. or greater per serving.

BRAND	ACCEPTABLE			NOT RECOMMENDED
	High fiber (3 grams or greater) no added fat	High fiber (3 grams or greater) contains acceptable oil (may be partially hydrogenated)	Low fiber or fiber content unknown, may contain acceptable oil (may be partially hydrogenated)	With added saturated fat
General Mills (Cont'd)	★Whole Grain Wheaties ★Whole Wheat Total		Kix Lucky charms Oatmeal crisp Oatmeal raisin crisp Oatmeal swirlers: ▽Apple cinnamon ▽Cherry ▽Strawberry Total corn flakes Triples ▽Trix	
Golden Harvest	Hot fiber cereal: ▽★Apples and cinnamon ▽★Maple and brown sugar ▽★Original flavor ▽★Oat bran ▽★Rice bran (15 grams fiber)			
Golden Temple			▽Cinnamon apple raisin granola ▽Lite n' crunchy granola	Coconut almond cereal Natural blueberry Super nutty granola

▽ Low sodium, 140 mg. or less per serving.
★ High fiber, 3 g. or greater per serving.

BRAND	ACCEPTABLE			NOT RECOMMENDED
	High fiber (3 grams or greater) no added fat	High fiber (3 grams or greater) contains acceptable oil (may be partially hydrogenated)	Low fiber or fiber content unknown, may contain acceptable oil (may be partially hydrogenated)	With added saturated fat
Grainfields	▽★Oat bran flakes ▽★Raisin bran ▽★Wheat flakes		▽Corn flakes ▽Crispy rice	

Health Valley	100% Natural bran cereal:
	  ▽★*Apples and cinnamon*
	  ▽★Raisin
	▽★*100% Natural cereal for babies*
	▽★*100% Natural stoned wheat raisin bran*
	▽★Blue corn flakes
	▽★Fruit and nut oat bran O's
	▽★Healthy O's
	▽★Oat bran
	Oat bran flakes:
	  ▽★Almonds, dates
	  ▽★Raisins
	  ▽★Regular
	Oat bran hot cereal:
	  ▽★Apples and cinnamon
	  ▽★Raisins and spice
		Orangeola:
		  ▽★Almonds and dates
		  ▽★*Bananas and Hawaiian fruit*
		Real oat bran cereal:
		  ▽★Almond crunch
		  ▽★Hawaiian fruit
		  ▽★Raisin nut
			Fruit lites:
			  ▽Brown rice
			  ▽Golden corn
			  ▽Golden wheat
			Raisin bran:
			  ▽Almonds and dates
			  ▽Regular
			Rice bran O's:
			  ▽Apple and cinnamon	

▽ Low sodium, 140 mg. or less per serving.
★ High fiber, 3 g. or greater per serving.

Brand	Acceptable			Not Recommended
	High fiber (3 grams or greater) no added fat	High fiber (3 grams or greater) contains acceptable oil (may be partially hydrogenated)	Low fiber or fiber content unknown, may contain acceptable oil (may be partially hydrogenated)	With added saturated fat
Health Valley (Cont'd)	Oat bran O's: ▽★Regular ▽★Sprouts 7 with raisins Swiss Breakfast: ▽★Raisin nut ▽★Tropical fruit ▽★Wheat germ and fiber with bananas and tropical fruit			
Hodgson Mills	▽★Bulgar wheat ▽★Cracked wheat cereal ▽★Oat bran ▽★Wheat bran (12 grams fiber) ▽★Wheat germ			
Kellogg's	★40% Bran flakes ★All bran (10 grams fiber) ▽★All bran with extra fiber (14 grams fiber) ★Apple raisin crisp ★Bran flakes Common Sense oat bran: ★Regular ★With raisins	Mueslix: ★Golden crunch apples and almonds	▽Apple Jacks Bigg Mixx: Plain Raisins Cinnamon mini buns Cocoa Krispies Corn flakes ▽Corn Pops Crispix Frosted flakes	Cracklin' oat bran Froot Loops Oatbake: Honey bran Raisin nut

▽ Low sodium, 140 mg. or less per serving.
★ High fiber, 3 g. or greater per serving.

BRAND	ACCEPTABLE			NOT RECOMMENDED
	High fiber (3 grams or greater) no added fat	High fiber (3 grams or greater) contains acceptable oil (may be partially hydrogenated)	Low fiber or fiber content unknown, may contain acceptable oil (may be partially hydrogenated)	With added saturated fat
Kellogg's (Cont'd)	Frosted Mini Wheats: 　▽★Bite size 　▽★Original size ★Fruitful bran ▽★Heartwise Mueslix: 　★Crispy blend, raisin, date and almond Nutri Grain: 　★Almond raisin 　▽★Biscuits 　★Raisin bran 　★Wheat ★Raisin bran S. W. Graham: 　★Plain Shredded wheat squares: 　▽★Strawberry		Fruity Marshmallow Krispies ▽Honey Smacks Just Right: 　Fiber nuggets 　Fruit and nuts Kenmei: 　Rice bran 　Rice bran with almonds and raisins Nut 'n Honey Crunch O's Nut 'n Honey Crunch Product 19 Rice Krispies S. W. Graham: 　Brown sugar and cinnamon Shredded wheat squares: 　▽Apple cinnamon 　▽Raisin Special K	
Kolln	▽★Crispy oats ▽★Fruit 'n oat bran crunch ▽★Oat bran crunch			

▽ Low sodium, 140 mg. or less per serving.
★ High fiber, 3 g. or greater per serving.

BRAND	ACCEPTABLE			NOT RECOMMENDED
	High fiber (3 grams or greater) no added fat	High fiber (3 grams or greater) contains acceptable oil (may be partially hydrogenated)	Low fiber or fiber content unknown, may contain acceptable oil (may be partially hydrogenated)	With added saturated fat
Kretschmer	▽★Wheat germ			
Kroger	▽★Oat bran ▽★Quick oats ★Raisin bran		Corn flakes Crispy rice Frosted flakes ▽Frosted wheat puffs ▽Fruit Rings Honey and Nut sweetened toasted oats Instant oatmeal: 　▽Apple and cinnamon 　Maple and brown sugar ▽Nutty Nuggets ▽Rice puffs Toasted oats ▽Wheat puffs	
Little Crow Foods	▽★CoCo Wheats			
Malt-O-Meal	▽★Quick Malt-O-Meal plus 40% oat bran		▽Quick Malt-O-Meal	
Nabisco	★100% Bran (10 grams fiber) ★100% Bran with oat bran		▽Cream of rice ▽Instant cream of wheat	

▽ Low sodium, 140 mg. or less per serving.
★ High fiber, 3 g. or greater per serving.

BRAND	ACCEPTABLE			NOT RECOMMENDED
	High fiber (3 grams or greater) no added fat	High fiber (3 grams or greater) contains acceptable oil (may be partially hydrogenated)	Low fiber or fiber content unknown, may contain acceptable oil (may be partially hydrogenated)	With added saturated fat
Nabisco (Cont'd)	▽★Frosted wheat squares Fruit wheats: 　▽★Raspberry Instant oat bran: 　★Apple cinnamon 　▽★Regular ▽★Oat bran ▽★Shredded wheat ▽★Shredded wheat 'n bran ★Shredded wheat with oat bran ▽★Spoon size shredded wheat		Instant Mix 'n Eat cream of wheat: 　Apple 'n cinnamon 　*Maple and brown sugar* 　Original ▽Quick cream of wheat Team flakes Teddy graham breakfast bears: 　▽Chocolate 　▽Cinnamon 　▽Honey	
Old Wessex Ltd.	▽★*Oat bran*			
Perky's			▽Crispy brown rice Nutty rice: 　▽Raisin sweetened	
Pet Inc.			▽Heartland Natural with raisins	
Post	★Bran flakes ★Grape-nuts ★Natural raisin bran	Fruit and Fibre: 　★Date, raisin, walnut and oat clusters	Alphabits: 　▽Marshmallow 　Regular	Cocoa Pebbles *Croonchy Stars*

▽ Low sodium, 140 mg. or less per serving.
★ High fiber, 3 g. or greater per serving.

BRAND	ACCEPTABLE			NOT RECOMMENDED
	High fiber (3 grams or greater) no added fat	High fiber (3 grams or greater) contains acceptable oil (may be partially hydrogenated)	Low fiber or fiber content unknown, may contain acceptable oil (may be partially hydrogenated)	With added saturated fat

Post (Cont'd)	★Raisin bran	★Grape-nut flakes	Fruity Pebbles
			Honey Bunches of Oats:
			  Almonds
			  Honey roasted
			Honey Comb
			▽Oat flakes
			▽Super Golden Crisp
			Toasties corn flakes
				Fruit and Fibre:
				  Cinnamon apple crisp
				  Pineapple, banana and coconut

Quaker	Instant oatmeal:
	  ▽★Apple and cinnamon
	  ★Cinnamon and spice
	  ★Maple and brown sugar
	  ★Regular
	Instant Quaker Extra:
	  ★Regular
	Mother's:
	  ▽★Instant oatmeal
	  ▽★Oat bran
	  ▽★Rolled oats
	  ▽★Whole wheat (hot natural cereal)
	  ▽★Oat bran
		Instant oatmeal:
		  ★Apple, raisin, walnut
		  ★Raisin and spice
		Instant Quaker Extra:
		  ▽★Raisins and cinnamon
		Oat bran hot cereal:
		  ▽★Raisin and cinnamon
			▽Apple Cinnamon Oh's
			Cinnamon Life
			Crunchy rice bran
			Honey Graham Oh's
			Instant grits
			Instant oatmeal:
			  Bananas and cream
			  Blueberries and cream
			  Honey nut
			  Peaches and cream
			  Strawberries and cream
			Instant Quaker Extra:
			  Apples and spice
			Life
			▽Puffed rice
				100% Natural cereal:
				  Raisin and date
				Cap'n Crunch
				Cap'n Crunch's Crunch Berries
				Cap'n Crunch's Peanut Butter
				Corn bran
				Crunchy bran
				Crunchy Nut Oh's
				King Vitamin

▽ Low sodium, 140 mg. or less per serving.
★ High fiber, 3 g. or greater per serving.

BRAND	ACCEPTABLE			NOT RECOMMENDED
	High fiber (3 grams or greater) no added fat	High fiber (3 grams or greater) contains acceptable oil (may be partially hydrogenated)	Low fiber or fiber content unknown, may contain acceptable oil (may be partially hydrogenated)	With added saturated fat

Quaker (Cont'd)	▽★Oat bran cereal
	Oat bran hot cereal:
	  ▽★Apple and spice
	▽★Old fashioned Quaker oats
	▽★Quick Quaker oats
	Rice bran:
	  ▽★Honey crunch
			▽Puffed wheat
			Quaker Oat Squares
			▽Quick grits
			▽Sun Country granola and almonds
			Tiny Toons	

Ralston	★*Bran Chex*
	Bran News:
	  ★Hint of Cinnamon
	▽★High fiber hot cereal
	★Multibran chex
		Muesli:
		  ▽★Raisins, dates, almonds
		  ▽★Raisins, peaches, pecans
		  ▽★Raisins, walnuts, cranberries
		★Oat Bran Options:
		Flakes with raisins, dates and oat nuggets
		Rice bran options:
		  ▽★Flakes with oat nuggets
			▽Batman
			Chocolate chip Cookie Crisp
			Corn Chex
			Double Chex
			Honey Graham Chex
			Hot wheels
			Rice Chex
			Teenage Mutant Ninja Turtles
			Wheat Chex
				Almond delight
				Morning Funnies
				Nintendo

Roman Meal	▽★Cream of rye			

Sovex	Instant oatmeal:
	  ▽★Apples and cinnamon
			Good Shepherd:
			  ▽Almonds and molasses
				Crunchy granola with added bran

▽ Low sodium, 140 mg. or less per serving.
★ High fiber, 3 g. or greater per serving.

BRAND	ACCEPTABLE			NOT RECOMMENDED
	High fiber (3 grams or greater) no added fat	High fiber (3 grams or greater) contains acceptable oil (may be partially hydrogenated)	Low fiber or fiber content unknown, may contain acceptable oil (may be partially hydrogenated)	With added saturated fat
Sovex (Cont'd)	Instant oatmeal (Cont'd): ▽★Maple and brown sugar ▽★Regular ▽★Oat bran		Good Shepherd (Cont'd): ▽Unsweetened ▽Honey almond granola	Fruit and nut granola Good Shepherd: Traditional Wheat free
Stone-Buhr	▽★7 Grain cereal ▽★Hot apple granola ▽★Untoasted wheat germ		▽Bran flakes	
Tree of Life	▽★*Oat bran*			
U.S. Mills	▽★Uncle Sam			
Weetabix	▽★Weetabix whole wheat cereal			

▽ Low sodium, 140 mg. or less per serving.
★ High fiber, 3 g. or greater per serving.

Pasta, Potato and Grain Mixes

ACCEPTABLE

■ **Whole grains, without added fat**

These products are preferred because they are the least processed and are made from whole grains. Fat has not been added in the processing, leaving that choice to you when you prepare the item at home.

■ **Refined grains or may contain acceptable oil or meat**

Items in this category are acceptable; however, the grains are refined and fat or eggs may have been added in the processing. Pasta made with eggs will be identified with a (•) symbol. Egg noodles contain 50-70 mg. cholesterol per 2 ounce serving (dry weight).

Although products in this section contain acceptable fat, they may also contain too much fat. To lower the fat content of prepared mixes, use skim milk and decrease by half or eliminate the fat called for on the package instructions.

NOT RECOMMENDED

■ **With added saturated fat**

Pasta, potato and grain mixes with added saturated fat are not recommended.

NOTE

■ The macaroni and cheese dinners are in the **NOT RECOMMENDED** column because they are processed with regular cheese. The products marked with an (*) asterisk can be prepared in a manner to make them acceptable and yield less than 30% fat calories. Simply modify the preparation directions by using skim milk and eliminating the margarine.

■ Many of these prepared mixes are high in sodium and can provide as much as 500-1700 mg. sodium per serving. To decrease the sodium content of these mixes, we suggest using approximately half of the seasoning packet that is normally provided for preparation. If additional seasonings are needed use fresh herbs or dried herbs prepared without salt. Sodium symbols are used to indicate high (▲) or low (▽) sodium **only** when sodium content is provided on the product label. Those products that are not identified with either symbol may be either high or low sodium or contain between 141-399 mg. sodium per serving.

BRAND	ACCEPTABLE		NOT RECOMMENDED
	Whole grains without added fat	Refined grains or may contain acceptable oil or meat	With added saturated fat
All brands	▽Brown rice Whole wheat: 　Lasagna 　Macaroni 　Spaghetti	•Alphabets Barley: 　▽Medium, fine, pearled Cavatelli Couscous •Egg noodles (all types) Elbows •Fettucini Instant rice •Kluski Lasagna Linguini Macaroni Mostaccioli Rice: 　All types (except brown and 　　wild) Rigatoni Shells Spaghetti Torroncini Vermicelli Ziti	
Amore			Tortellini with cheese: 　Plain 　*Spinach*
Arrowhead Mills	▽Quick brown rice		

▽ Low sodium, 140 mg. or less per serving.
• Contains egg yolks.

BRAND	ACCEPTABLE		NOT RECOMMENDED
	Whole grains without added fat	Refined grains or may contain acceptable oil or meat	With added saturated fat
Barbara's		▽Mashed potatoes	
Bascom's	100% wild rice		
Betty Crocker		Hamburger Helper: ▲*Chili* ▲*Chili and beans* ▲Chili tomato ▽Hash brown potatoes ▽Potato Buds mashed potatoes ▲Scalloped 'n Ham potatoes Suddenly Salad: ▲Classic pasta Creamy macaroni	Au gratin potatoes Cheddar 'n Bacon potatoes Chicken Helper: *Chicken and stuffing* Hamburger Helper: Beef noodle Cheeseburger macaroni Cheesy Italian Hamburger potatoes au gratin Lasagna Meatloaf Stroganoff Julienne potatoes Microwave potatoes: *Creamy scalloped* *Mild cheddar cheese* *Rich sour cream* Potato medleys: *Broccoli au gratin* *Cheddar cheese with mushrooms* *Scalloped with broccoli* *Scalloped with green beans and mushrooms*

▲ High sodium, 400 mg. or greater per serving.
▽ Low sodium, 140 mg. or less per serving.

BRAND	ACCEPTABLE		NOT RECOMMENDED
	Whole grains without added fat	Refined grains or may contain acceptable oil or meat	With added saturated fat
Betty Crocker (Cont'd)			Scalloped potatoes Smokey cheddar flavored potatoes Sour cream 'n chive potatoes Suddenly Salad: _Caesar_ Ranch and bacon _Tortellini Italiano_ Tuna Helper: _Buttery rice_ Cheesy noodles _Creamy mushroom and tuna_ Creamy noodles Fettuccine Alfredo _Tuna pot pie_ Twice baked family style potatoes: Bacon and cheddar
Buitoni		High protein pasta: ▽Linguine ▽Mostaccioli riguti ▽Rich spinach flavor shells ▽Rigatoni ▽Spinach linguine ▽Thin spaghetti ▽Vermicelli	

▽ Low sodium, 140 mg. or less per serving.

BRAND	ACCEPTABLE		NOT RECOMMENDED
	Whole grains without added fat	Refined grains or may contain acceptable oil or meat	With added saturated fat
Chef Boyardee		Hamburger Italiano: 　Hearty lasagna 　Pizza spirals 　Shells robusto	
Cost Cutter		▽•Egg noodles ▽Elbow macaroni ▽Spaghetti	*Macaroni and cheese dinner
Creamette		▽•Dumpling egg noodles (70 mg. cholesterol/serving) ▽•Egg noodles (70 mg. cholesterol/serving) Lasagna Macaroni ▽Mostaccioli *Rainbow rotini* Ribbons: 　▽Plain 　▽Spinach ▽Rotelle ▽Rotini ▽Spaghetti	
DaVinci		▽Fusilli springs ▽Rigatoni ▽Rotelle wagon wheels ▽Spaghetti	

▽ Low sodium, 140 mg. or less per serving.
• Contains egg yolks.
* This product can be made acceptable by modifying preparation methods to use skim milk and eliminate adding margarine.

BRAND	ACCEPTABLE		NOT RECOMMENDED
	Whole grains without added fat	**Refined grains or may contain acceptable oil or meat**	**With added saturated fat**
DaVinci (Cont'd)		▽Spinach nests Tortellini: 　▲•*Multi-color* 　▲•Plain 　▲•Ravioletti 　▲•Spinach	
DeBole's	▽Whole wheat spaghetti	▽Eggless noodles ▽*Pasta primavera vegetable shells* Pasta substitute: 　▽Angel hair pasta 　▽Curly lasagna 　▽Eggless noodles 　▽Fettuccini 　▽Linguine 　▽Rotini 　▽Spinach fettuccini 　▽Spinach spaghetti 　▽Thin spaghetti	*Macaroni and cheese dinner *Noodles and cheese dinner* *Whole wheat macaroni and cheese dinner*
Eden		▽Paella ribbons with saffron ▽Parsley garlic ribbons	
Fantastic Foods		Couscous Tabouli salad mix	
Gibbs	▽Wild rice		

▲ High sodium, 400 mg. or greater per serving.
▽ Low sodium, 140 mg. or less per serving.
• Contains egg yolks.
* This product can be made acceptable by modifying preparation methods to use skim milk and eliminate adding margarine.

BRAND	ACCEPTABLE		NOT RECOMMENDED
	Whole grains without added fat	Refined grains or may contain acceptable oil or meat	With added saturated fat

Golden Grain		Noodle Roni:
		▲*Broccoli and mushroom*
		Parmesano
		Rice-a-Roni:
		▲Beef
		▲Fried rice
		▲Long grain and wild rice
		▲Spanish rice
			*Macaroni and cheddar
			Noodle Roni:
			  Chicken and mushroom flavor
			  Creamy chicken
			  Fettucine
			  Mild cheddar
			  Vegetable alfredo
			Rice-a-Roni:
			  Beef and mushroom
			  Chicken
			  Chicken and broccoli
			  Chicken and mushroom
			  Chicken and vegetables
			  Chicken with almonds
			  Rice pilaf
			Rice-a-Roni Savory Classics:
			  Broccoli au gratin
			  Chicken Florentine
			  Creamy parmesan and herbs
			  Garden pilaf
			  Green bean almondine

Goodman's		▽•Alphabets, enriched egg noodles	
Greenfield's		▽•Eggdrop farfel ▽•Extra fine egg noodles	

▲ High sodium, 400 mg. or greater per serving.
▽ Low sodium, 140 mg. or less per serving.
• Contains egg yolks.
* This product can be made acceptable by modifying preparation methods to use skim milk and eliminate adding margarine.

BRAND	ACCEPTABLE		NOT RECOMMENDED
	Whole grains without added fat	**Refined grains or may contain acceptable oil or meat**	**With added saturated fat**
Greenfield's (Cont'd)		Homemade style egg noodles: ▽•Bow ties ▽•Extra wide	

Hain	Hain Naturals:
	  Chicken meatless style
	  ▲Herb
	  Rice almondine
	Pasta and sauce:
	  Italian herb
			Pasta and sauce:
			  Creamy Swiss
			  Fettucine Alfredo
			  Tangy cheddar

Health Valley	▽Whole wheat pasta ▽Whole wheat spinach pasta		

Hodgson Mills	Whole wheat pasta:
	  ▽•Egg noodles
	  ▽Fettuccine
	  ▽Lasagna
	  ▽Spaghetti
	  ▽Spinach spaghetti
		▽Veggie rotini	*Whole wheat macaroni and cheese

Hunt's		Minute Gourmet:
		  ▲Chicken cacciatore
		  Chicken with long grain wild rice
		  Potato stroganoff
		  Sweet and sour chicken
			Minute Gourmet:
			  Oriental beef
			  Pasta beef stroganoff dinner

▲ High sodium, 400 mg. or greater per serving.
▽ Low sodium, 140 mg. or less per serving.
• Contains egg yolks.
* This product can be made acceptable by modifying preparation methods to use skim milk and eliminate adding margarine.

BRAND	ACCEPTABLE		NOT RECOMMENDED
	Whole grains without added fat	Refined grains or may contain acceptable oil or meat	With added saturated fat

International Bazaar	▽Extra fancy wild rice
	Long grain brown and wild rice:
	  Beef flavor
			Long grain and wild rice:
			  Chicken flavor and herbs

Jane's			*Krazy mixed up rice*
Konriko	Cajun rice pilaf Wild pecan rice		

Kraft		Pasta salad:
		  Garden primavera
		  •*Homestyle*
			Deluxe macaroni and cheese
			Egg noodle with chicken dinner
			Macaroni and cheese:
			  *Music mac
			  *Regular
			  *Spirals
			  *Wheels
			Pasta and cheese:
			  Cheddar broccoli
			  Fettuccine alfredo
			  Herb and garlic
			  Parmesan
			Pasta salad:
			  Ranchers choice with bacon
			Potatoes and cheese:
			  Au gratin
			  Broccoli au gratin
			  Scalloped

▽ Low sodium, 140 mg. or less per serving.
• Contains egg yolks.
* This product can be made acceptable by modifying preparation methods to use skim milk and eliminate adding margarine.

BRAND	ACCEPTABLE		NOT RECOMMENDED
	Whole grains without added fat	Refined grains or may contain acceptable oil or meat	With added saturated fat

Kraft (Cont'd)			Rice and cheese:
			    Cheddar broccoli
			    Cheddar chicken
			    Cheddar pilaf

Kroger		▽•Egg noodles (all sizes)
		▽Elbow macaroni
		Hamburger Magic:
		    ▲Beefy rice
		    ▲•Chili tomato
		    ▲•Lasagna
		    ▲Pan pizza
		    ▲Taco casserole
		▽Instant enriched pre-cooked rice
		▽Instant mashed potatoes
		▽Lasagna
		▲Long grain and wild rice
		Noodle Magic:
		    •Chicken flavor
		Potato Magic:
		    Sour cream and chives
		▽*Rainbow salad twirls*
		▽*Salad bows*
		Salad Magic:
		    Classic pasta
		    Italian pasta
			Au gratin potatoes
			Hamburger Magic:
			    Beefy noodle
			    Cheeseburger macaroni
			    Potato stroganoff
			Macaroni and cheese dinner
			Noodle Magic:
			    Beef flavor
			Potato Magic:
			    Cheddar and bacon
			    Cheddar and mushrooms
			    Green beans and mushrooms
			Salad Magic:
			    Broccoli au gratin
			    Creamy macaroni
			Scalloped potatoes
			Tuna Magic:
			    Noodles and cheese sauce
			    Noodles and cream sauce

▲ High sodium, 400 mg. or greater per serving.
▽ Low sodium, 140 mg. or less per serving.
• Contains egg yolks.

BRAND	ACCEPTABLE		NOT RECOMMENDED
	Whole grains without added fat	Refined grains or may contain acceptable oil or meat	With added saturated fat
Kroger (Cont'd)		▽*Salad rotini* ▽Salad shells ▽Spaghetti	

Light n' Fluffy		Egg noodles (55 mg. cholesterol/serving):
		    ▽•Plain
		    •Spinach
		▽Macaroni dumplings
		▽Rainbow Twirls	

Lipton		Rice and beans:
		    ▲Chicken flavor
		Rice and sauce:
		    ▲Cajun style
		    ▲Mushroom
		    ▲*Rice Cajun-style*
		    ▲Spanish
			Long grain and wild rice:
			    Original recipe
			Noodles and sauce:
			    Alfredo
			    Butter
			    Chicken
			    Sour cream and chives
			    Stroganoff
			Pasta and sauce:
			    Cheddar broccoli
			    Creamy garlic
			Rice and sauce:
			    Broccoli and cheddar cheese
			    Chicken
			    Long grain and wild rice
			    Rice broccoli

▲ High sodium, 400 mg. or greater per serving.
▽ Low sodium, 140 mg. or less per serving.
• Contains egg yolks.

BRAND	ACCEPTABLE		NOT RECOMMENDED
	Whole grains without added fat	Refined grains or may contain acceptable oil or meat	With added saturated fat
Luzianne		▲Etouffee dinner ▲Gumbo dinner ▲Jambalaya dinner ▲Shrimp creole dinner	
Maggi		•Spaetzle	
Martha White		Spud flakes instant mashed potatoes	
Minute		Rice: ▽Natural long grain ▽Original ▽Premium long grain rice	
Minute Microwave			Cheddar cheese, broccoli and rice Chicken flavored noodles Chicken flavored rice Noodles alfredo Parmesan noodles Pasta and cheddar cheese
Mother's	▽Quick Cooking Barley		
Mrs. Weiss		Egg noodles: ▽•Plain (thin and wide) •Rainbow ▽•Spinach ▽•Kluski egg noodle dumpling	

▲ High sodium, 400 mg. or greater per serving.
▽ Low sodium, 140 mg. or less per serving.
• Contains egg yolks.

BRAND	ACCEPTABLE		NOT RECOMMENDED
	Whole grains without added fat	Refined grains or may contain acceptable oil or meat	With added saturated fat

Mueller's		▽●Hearty egg noodles
		▽●Kluski
		▽Lasagna
		▽Macaroni
		▽●Old fashioned egg noodles (all sizes)
		▽Pasta frills
		▽Pasta ruffles
		▽*Ruffle trio*
		Salad bar pasta:
		  Pasta classico
		▽Sea shells
		▽Spaghetti
		▽*Spring trio*
		▽Super shapes
		▽Twist trio
		▽Vermicelli
			Chef's Series:
			  Alfredo
			  Chicken flavor
			  Stroganoff

Natural		▽Superoni elbows ▽Superoni thin spaghetti	

Near East	Taboule wheat salad mix
	Wheat pilaf mix
		▽Couscous Moroccan pasta
		Rice pilaf mix:
		  ▲Beef flavor
		  ▲Regular
		▲Spanish rice mix
			Rice pilaf mix:
			  Chicken flavor

No Yolks		▽Cholesterol free egg noodle substitute (all sizes)	

▲ High sodium, 400 mg. or greater per serving.
▽ Low sodium, 140 mg. or less per serving.
● Contains egg yolks.

BRAND	ACCEPTABLE		NOT RECOMMENDED
	Whole grains without added fat	Refined grains or may contain acceptable oil or meat	With added saturated fat
Panni		Potato dumpling mix: Bavarian Shredded potato Potato pancake mix: Bavarian Shredded potato	
Perfection		Microwave pasta: Elbows Mostaccioli Small rigatoni	
Pillsbury		▽Hungry Jack instant mashed potatoes	Real cheese sauce scalloped potatoes Tangy au gratin potatoes
Primera			*Turtles and cheese pasta dinner
Prince		▽Alphabets ▽Curly lasagna Dutch Maid egg noodles: ▽•Broad ▽•Country style ▽•Wide ▽•Egg noodle bows ▽•Egg noodle flakes ▽•Egg pastina ▽Elbows Folded fettuccine: ▽•Egg noodle product	

▽ Low sodium, 140 mg. or less per serving.
• Contains egg yolks.
* This product can be made acceptable by modifying preparation methods to use skim milk and eliminate adding margarine.

Brand	Acceptable		Not Recommended
	Whole grains without added fat	Refined grains or may contain acceptable oil or meat	With added saturated fat

Prince (Cont'd)		▽Light elbows
		▽Linguine
		▽Manicotti
		▽Mostacciolini
		▽Orzo
		▽Rigatoni
		▽Rotini
		▽Rotini primavera
		▽Shells (all sizes)
		▽*Shells primavera*
		Silver Award:
		  ▽•Fettucine
		  ▽Linguine Pomodoro e Basilico
		  ▽•Paglia e Fieno
		  ▽Penne all' Arrabbiata
		    (mostaccioli)
		▽Soup-mac
		▽Spaghetti
		▽•Spinach egg noodles
		▽*Superoni elbows*
		▽Torroncini
		▽Vermicelli
		▽Yolk-free egg noodle substitute	

Pritikin	▽Whole wheat spaghetti		
Quaker	▽Quick barley		
R.M. Quigg's		Golden mix: Curry rice	

▽ Low sodium, 140 mg. or less per serving.
• Contains egg yolks.

BRAND	ACCEPTABLE		NOT RECOMMENDED
	Whole grains without added fat	Refined grains or may contain acceptable oil or meat	With added saturated fat
R.M. Quigg's (Cont'd)		Golden mix (Cont'd): French onion Herb rice Paella rice Ranch rice Yellow rice	
Riceland	▽Natural brown rice		
Riviana		▽Success rice	
San Giorgio		▽Alphabets ▽Cut fusilli ▽Cut ziti ▽Ditalini ▽•Fettuccine (55 mg. cholesterol/serving) ▽Lasagna ▽Linguine ▽Manicotti ▽Rotelle ▽Rotini ▽Shells (all sizes) ▽Vermicelli	
Suzi Wan		*Sweet 'n sour* *Teriyaki*	
Texmati	▽Brown rice	▽Royal blend with wild rice	

▽ Low sodium, 140 mg. or less per serving.
• Contains egg yolks.

BRAND	ACCEPTABLE		NOT RECOMMENDED
	Whole grains without added fat	Refined grains or may contain acceptable oil or meat	With added saturated fat

Uncle Ben's	▽Fast cooking whole grain brown rice
	▽Instant brown rice
	▽Natural whole grain rice
		▽Boil-in-bag rice
		Converted rice:
		  ▽Natural long grain
		▽Enriched white rice
		Fast cooking long grain and wild rice:
		    ▲Original
		Long grain and wild rice:
		    ▲Original recipe and 23 herbs and seasonings
		▽Rice in an Instant
			Country Inn rice:
			  Broccoli almondine
			  Broccoli rice au gratin
			  Cauliflower au gratin
			  Chicken and cheese Risotto
			  Chicken rice royale
			  Chicken stock rice with pasta shells
			  Homestyle chicken and vegetable
			  Rice Alfredo
			  Veg. medley
			Fast cooking long grain and wild rice:
			    Chicken stock sauce with vegetables

Velveeta			Shells and cheese dinner
Vigo		Yellow rice	Risotto con broccoli
Voyager		Curry rice French onion Herb rice Long grain and wild rice *Spanish rice*	
Worthington	▲Grain burger		

▲ High sodium, 400 mg. or greater per serving.
▽ Low sodium, 140 mg. or less per serving.

LEGUMES

Legumes include a wide variety of dry beans and peas. They are excellent sources of complex carbohydrate (starch), fiber, protein, potassium, phosphorous and iron. When legumes are combined with grains such as rice, wheat, barley, corn or oats, the quality of protein they provide is equally as complete as that of meat or dairy products. Additionally, legumes contain no cholesterol and only minimal amounts of saturated fat. They are also high in water-soluble fiber which has been shown to help lower cholesterol levels and to stabilize blood sugar.

Because of the excellent nutritional quality and health benefits that legumes provide, regular consumption is recommended. Soaking beans overnight shortens the cooking time by tenderizing the beans. Soaking also enhances digestibility by reducing the substances (oligosaccharides) that cause flatulence (gas). To further enhance digestibility, it is recommended that the soaking water be discarded and replaced with fresh water before cooking.

TYPES OF BEANS AND THEIR PREPARATION TIME

Types of Beans	Soaking	Cooking	Pressure Cooking Soaking	Pressure Cooking Cooking
Soft Beans Lentils Mung Beans Split Peas Black-eyed Peas	None	1-2 hrs	none	45 min
Medium Beans Azuki, Pinto, Kidney, Navy, Lima, Black, Turtle	2-4 hrs	2 hrs	1 hr	1 hr
Hard Beans Garbanzo (chick peas) Soybeans	6-8 hrs or overnight	4 hrs	2 hrs	1-2 hrs

Tips for Bean Cuisine:

Storage: Store in airtight containers in a cool, dark place.

Yield: 1 cup dried beans (1/2 lb.) = 2 cups cooked beans.

Soaking:

- Always sort and wash beans before soaking.
- See chart for soaking times. You may also use the "quick soak" method. Bring water and beans to a boil; let boil for 1-2 minutes, then let beans soak for two hours. This method reduces soaking time by 25%.

Eliminating the "infamous effect" of beans:

- Soak beans for 4-5 hours or overnight. Discard soaking water.
- Try sprouting beans before cooking.
- Add a 3-6" piece of KOMBU* (sea vegetable, available at health food stores or oriental food stores) to beans during cooking.
- Cook beans slowly and thoroughly.
- Eat small amounts of beans regularly at first, then increase consumption as tolerance increases.
- Begin by eating beans which cause less gas (e.g., lentils, black-eyed peas, limas, garbanzo beans [chick peas], white beans, tofu and tempeh).

Solving cooking problems:

- Plan meals one day ahead and pre-soak beans the night before or in the morning.
- On busy days, use beans which do not need to be soaked (e.g., lentils, split peas, mung).
- Buy already-cooked beans in jars or cans (watch labels!)
- Cook ahead; you may refrigerate beans for several days.
- Cook a double batch and freeze cooked beans for future use.

Seasoning:

- Avoid high fat pork products such as salt pork; instead try miso (soy, barley or rice). Miso is a fermented product, available in the health food sections of most grocery stores.

Kombu should be avoided by individuals sensitive to iodine.

Legumes

■ **Dried, unprocessed**

These products are preferred because they are whole, unprocessed and have had nothing added to them. This is also the most economical way to buy legumes. The only disadvantage is that these products take more time to prepare. (See page 211 for cooking tips.)

■ **Processed without added fat**

These products are more convenient because they have already been cooked. The disadvantage to these products is that sodium, and in many cases sugar and preservatives, have been added in processing. Therefore, it is best to rinse canned beans before using. When preparing dry bean mixes, decrease or eliminate the oil that is called for on the package instructions.

■ **Processed with added acceptable oil or meat**

These products are also acceptable, convenient food choices, but are higher in fat because oil has been used in processing.

NOT RECOMMENDED

■ **Processed with added saturated fat**

Products with added saturated fat should be avoided.

NOTE

■ There is a wide range of sodium content for foods in this category. Dry, unprocessed beans cooked without salt are very low in sodium containing approximately 3 mg. per ½ cup serving. On the other hand, canned beans can contain as much as 300-500 mg. per ½ cup serving. Sodium symbols are used to indicate high (▲) or low (▽) sodium **only** when sodium content is provided on the product label. Those products that are not identified with either symbol may be either high or low sodium or contain between 141-399 mg. sodium per serving.

BRAND	ACCEPTABLE			NOT RECOMMENDED
	Dried, unprocessed	Processed without added fat	Processed with added acceptable oil or meat	Processed with added saturated fat
All brands	★Black beans ★Garbanzo beans ★Great northern beans ★Lentils ★Michigan navy beans ★Minestrone soup mix (beans only) ★Red kidney beans ★Soy beans ★Yellow split peas			Pork and beans
B & M				Brick oven baked beans
Brooks		▲★Chili hot beans ▲Chili mix		
Bush's Best		★Dark red kidney beans ▲★Deluxe vegetarian beans	★Chili hot beans	Baked beans: 　Bacon 　Onions Deluxe Pork & Beans
Campbell's		★Beans 'n Beef	▲★B B Q beans	Homestyle beans Old fashioned beans Pork and beans
Casa Fiesta				Refried beans
Casbah		★Hummus bean dip		
El Ebro				Black beans: 　Cuban style

▲ High sodium, 400 mg. or greater per serving.
★ High fiber, 3 g. or greater per serving.

BRAND	ACCEPTABLE			NOT RECOMMENDED
	Dried, unprocessed	Processed without added fat	Processed with added acceptable oil or meat	Processed with added saturated fat
El Rio		★Garbanzo beans ★Mexican beans		Refried beans
Fantastic Foods		Falafel mix ▲★Fantastic Jumpin' Black Beans ▲★Fantastic Splittin' Peas Nature's Burger Tofu burger Tofu scrambler	▲★Fantastic Cha-Cha Chili with beans ★*Instant black beans* ★Instant refried beans	
Fontova			★Refried beans with zesty mole sauce	
Frito Lay				Bean dip
Hain			★Hot bean dip ★*Natural jalapeño bean dip* ★Natural onion bean dip ★Vegetarian refried beans	
Hanover				Barbecue baked beans Brown sugar and bacon baked beans
Harvest Earth Foods			▽★Tempeh Delites	

▲ High sodium, 400 mg. or greater per serving.
▽ Low sodium, 140 mg. or less per serving.
★ High fiber, 3 g. or greater per serving.

BRAND	ACCEPTABLE			NOT RECOMMENDED
	Dried, unprocessed	Processed without added fat	Processed with added acceptable oil or meat	Processed with added saturated fat
Health Valley			Vegetarian chili with beans: 　▽★Mild 　★Spicy	
Heinz		▲★Vegetarian beans in tomato sauce		
Hunt's		Manwich: 　▲Chili fixin's		Big John's Beans 'n Fixins
Joan of Arc		★Fancy dark red kidney beans		
Kroger		▲★Bar-B-Q beans ▲★Beans with onions ▲★Great northern beans ★Kidney beans ▲★Pinto beans ▲★Red beans	▲★Country style beans in molasses sauce with pork ★*Jalapeño bean dip*	Baked beans with brown sugar and bacon Mexican style refried beans Pork and beans Texas beans
La Preferida		★Garbanzos/chick peas ★Pinto beans ★Pinto beans and jalapeños		Refried beans: 　Ranchero style 　Regular 　With sausage
La Victoria				Refried beans
Libby's				Deepbrown Pork and Beans: 　*In molasses sauce* 　*In tomato sauce*

▲ High sodium, 400 mg. or greater per serving.
▽ Low sodium, 140 mg. or less per serving.
★ High fiber, 3 g. or greater per serving.

BRAND	ACCEPTABLE			NOT RECOMMENDED
	Dried, unprocessed	Processed without added fat	Processed with added acceptable oil or meat	Processed with added saturated fat
Little Bear Organic Foods			Refried beans: ▽★No salt added ★Regular	
Near East		Falafel mix: ▲Vegetable burger mix Lentil pilaf mix		
Old El Paso				Jalapeño bean dip Refried beans: Regular with Cheese with Sausage
Ortega				Refried beans
Progresso		★Red kidney beans		
Randall		★Great northern beans ★Mixed beans ★Pinto beans		
S & W		★Chili Makins ★Maple sugar beans	★All-natural baked beans	Chili beans Smokey ranch beans
Seaside		★Chick peas garbanzos ★Dark red kidney beans		
Snack Time			★Jalapeño bean dip	
Taste Adventure		▲★Black bean flakes ▲★Pinto bean flakes ★Split Pea Soup		

▲ High sodium, 400 mg. or greater per serving.
★ High fiber, 3 g. or greater per serving.
▽ Low sodium, 140 mg. or less per serving.

BRAND	ACCEPTABLE			NOT RECOMMENDED
	Dried, unprocessed	Processed without added fat	Processed with added acceptable oil or meat	Processed with added saturated fat
Van deCamps		▲★Dark red kidney beans		Beanee Weanee: Beans with sliced hotdogs Pork and beans
Worthington		▲Vegetable scallops	▲Choplets ▲Fri Chik ▲Superlinks Vega links	

▲ High sodium, 400 mg. or greater per serving.
★ High fiber, 3 g. or greater per serving.

MEATS

This section contains listings with criteria for evaluating the following food categories:

◇ Beef, Lamb, Pork, and Veal
◇ Fish
◇ Poultry and Game
◇ Lunchmeats

Foods in the meat section are especially good sources of complete proteins, iron, zinc, vitamin B-12, niacin, potassium, phosphorous and other minerals. Some meats are also very rich sources of saturated fat and cholesterol. Therefore, it is recommended that you select lean meats most often, limit your intake of medium fat meats and avoid all high fat meats. In addition, your consumption of all red meats (i.e., beef, veal, lamb, pork) should be limited to 4 oz. three times per week. The majority of your meat consumption should come from fish, skinless white meat poultry or select species of wild game. Remember to trim all visible fat before cooking. When preparing meats, it is recommended that you bake, broil, grill or stir-fry using a small amount of monounsaturated oil (see pages 111-114), rather than deep fat fry.

NOTE
Most Americans can obtain adequate protein by consuming 6 ounces of meat, fish or poultry per day since many other foods also contain protein. Limiting your intake of all meats helps you to reduce the saturated fat and cholesterol content of your diet.

Beef, Lamb, Pork, Veal

ACCEPTABLE

▪ **Lean, less than 3 grams fat per ounce, trimmed**
Meats listed in this category are the leanest. Be sure to note the grade of meat when making your selections. Although meats in this category are the leanest, remember that they are still **red** meats and usually contain high levels of saturated fat.

▪ **Medium fat, between 3-5 grams fat per ounce, trimmed (select less often)**
Meats listed in this category are higher in fat and should be used less often than lean meats (i.e., those containing less than 3 grams fat per ounce). Remember that all meats should be skinned or trimmed of all visible fat before cooking.

NOT RECOMMENDED

▪ **High fat, greater than 5 grams fat per oz.**
These choices contain substantial amounts of fat and cholesterol and are not recommended.

NOTE

■ **All red meats contain higher levels of saturated fat than fish or poultry and should be limited to 4 ounces, three times per week (12 ounces per week).**

■ Organ meats such as kidney, sweet breads, liver and heart are high in cholesterol (e.g., liver contains 330 mg. per 3 ounce portion). It is recommended that you avoid all organ meats or consume them infrequently (i.e., limit to 4-6 ounces per month).

■ All fresh meat is low in sodium containing approximately 15-20 mg. sodium per ounce. Cured meats such as ham are much higher in sodium and contain approximately 250-300 mg. sodium per ounce. Fresh meats do not usually provide nutrition labeling; therefore, sodium symbols are not used in this section.

BRAND	ACCEPTABLE		NOT RECOMMENDED
	Lean, less than 3 grams fat per oz., trimmed	**Medium fat, between 3-5 grams fat per oz., trimmed (select less often)**	**High fat, greater than 5 grams fat per oz.**

Beef	Choice and select grades:
	  Chuck, arm pot roast
	  Round, bottom cut
	  Round, eye of round
	  Round, full cut
	  Round, tip round
	  Round, top round
	  Shortloin, tenderloin
	  Shortloin, top loin
	  Wedge-bone sirloin
	Choice grade:
	  Shank crosscuts
	  Shortloin, T-bone steak
	Lunchmeats and cured meats:
	  **Dried beef
	  Chopped beef
	  **Thin sliced beef
	Prime grade:
	  Round, Eye of round
	  Round, tip round
	  Round, top round
	Select grade:
	  Ribs, small end
		Choice and select grades:
		  Chuck, blade roast
		  Ribs, large end
		  Ribs, whole
		Choice grade:
		  Flank
		  Rib eye, small end
		  Ribs, small end
		  Shortloin, porterhouse steak
		Ground beef:
		  *Extra lean
		Prime grade:
		  Chuck, arm pot roast
		  Ribs, small end
		  Round, bottom round
		  Shortloin, tenderloin
		  Shortloin, top loin
		  Wedge-bone sirloin
			All prime cuts, unless otherwise indicated
			Choice grade:
			  Rib, short ribs
			Ground beef:
			  *Hamburger
			  *Lean
			  *Patties
			  *Regular
			Lunchmeats and cured meats:
			  **Beer salami
			  **Bologna
			  **Breakfast strips
			  **Corned beef brisket
			  **Frankfurter
			  **Pastrami
			  **Salami
			  **Sausage

*Since the fat content of 'ground beef' is not regulated by the U.S. Department of Agriculture, the amount of saturated fat in 'ground beef' varies from state to state.
**See pages 255-259 for specific lunchmeat brands.

BRAND	ACCEPTABLE		NOT RECOMMENDED
	Lean, less than 3 grams fat per oz., trimmed	Medium fat, between 3-5 grams fat per oz., trimmed (select less often)	High fat, greater than 5 grams fat per oz.
Beefalo	Beefalo: All parts		

Lamb	Choice grade:
	  Cubes, for stew
	  Foreshank
	  Leg, shank half
	  Leg, sirloin half
	  Leg, whole
	  Loin
		Choice grade:
		  Rib
		  Shoulder, arm
		  Shoulder, blade
		  Shoulder, whole
			Ground lamb

Pork	Canadian bacon
	Loin, tenderloin
	Lunchmeats and cured meats:
	  Ham steak, boneless, extra lean
	  Ham, boneless, extra lean
	  Ham, boneless, regular
	  Ham, center slice, country-style
	  Ham, whole
		Leg (ham), rump half
		Leg (ham), shank half
		Leg (ham), whole
		Loin, center loin
		Loin, center rib
		Loin, sirloin
		Loin, top loin
		Loin, whole
		Lunchmeats and cured meats:
		  Olive loaf
		Pigs feet
		Shoulder, arm picnic
		Shoulder, whole
			Bacon
			Bratwurst
			Braunschweiger
			Loin, blade
			Lunchmeats and cured meats:
			  **Beer salami
			  **Bologna
			  **Breakfast strips
			  **Salami, dry or hard
			  Ham and cheese loaf
			**Sausage
			Shoulder, blade, Boston
			Spare ribs

**See pages 255-259 for specific lunchmeat brands.

BRAND	ACCEPTABLE		NOT RECOMMENDED
	Lean, less than 3 grams fat per oz., trimmed	Medium fat, between 3-5 grams fat per oz., trimmed (select less often)	High fat, greater than 5 grams fat per oz.
Veal	Cubes, for stew Ground veal Leg (top round) Loin Rib Shoulder, arm Shoulder, blade Sirloin		

Fish

All types of fish are acceptable and should be eaten regularly. Fish selections are listed according to their Omega-3 fatty acids:

■ **Moderate to high in Omega-3 fatty acids, greater than or equal to 1 gram per 3.5 oz.**

■ **Lower in Omega-3 fatty acids, less than 1 gram per 3.5 oz.**

Like meat, fish and shellfish are good sources of complete proteins, vitamins and minerals; but **unlike** meat they are low in fat and particularly low in saturated fat. More importantly, some fish are high in a type of polyunsaturated fat called Omega-3 fatty acids.

Omega-3 fatty acids are thought to protect against heart disease in three ways: (1) by thinning the blood, making platelets less sticky and, therefore, less likely to cause a blood clot; (2) by lowering blood triglycerides; and (3) by decreasing the tendency of white blood cells to stick to the linings of arteries, thereby inhibiting the incorporation of fat into the walls of the arteries.

At this time it is not known how much Omega-3 fatty acids are needed in order to have a beneficial effect. However, research has shown that men who eat as little as 8 ounces of fish per week are half as likely to die from heart disease as those who do not eat fish.[45] It is recommended that you eat at least 8 ounces of fish per week.

NOTE

■ Fish oil capsules or supplements to lower blood cholesterol levels are not recommended. Health risks of taking fish oil supplements may include:
  • undesirable effects on blood clotting
  • possible toxic amounts of vitamins A and D
  • possible presence of environmental contaminants such as lead or mercury
  • possible increased vitamin requirements.

- Newer, more sophisticated analytical methods for measuring the cholesterol content of shellfish have revealed that shellfish are lower in cholesterol than previously thought. Most shellfish (e.g., lobster, clams, oysters, scallops, and crab), on average, contain lower amounts of cholesterol than equal portions of lean red meats or poultry. Although shrimp contains twice the amount of cholesterol as equal portions of lean meats, it is 91% lower in saturated fat. As discussed on page 8, saturated fat elevates blood cholesterol more than dietary cholesterol. Therefore, shrimp can be included as part of a low cholesterol, low saturated fat diet.

- When preparing fish, it is recommended to bake, broil or poach rather than fry.

- The sodium content of fresh fish is approximately 15-20 mg. per ounce. Fresh fish does not usually provide nutrient labeling; therefore, sodium symbols are not used in this section.

ACCEPTABLE	RECOMMEND AT LEAST 8 OZ. PER WEEK	
	Moderate to high in Omega-3 fatty acids, greater than or equal to 1 gram per 3.5 oz.	Lower in Omega-3 fatty acids, less than 1 gram per 3.5 oz.
Crustaceans		Crab, Alaska king Crab, blue Crab, Dungeness Crab, queen Crayfish, unspecified Lobster, European Lobster, northern Shrimp, Atlantic brown Shrimp, Atlantic white Shrimp, Japanese Shrimp, northern Shrimp, other Spiny lobster, Caribbean Spiny lobster, southern rock
Finfish	Anchovy Bluefish Capelin Dogfish, spiny Herring, Atlantic Herring, Pacific Herring, round Mackerel, Atlantic Mackerel, chub Mackerel, Japanese horse Mackerel, king Mullet, unspecified Sablefish Salmon, Atlantic Salmon, chinook	Bass, freshwater Bass, striped Burbot Carp Catfish, brown Catfish, channel Cisco Cod, Atlantic Cod, Pacific Croaker, Atlantic Dolphinfish Drum, black Drum, freshwater Eel, European Flounder, unspecified

ACCEPTABLE	RECOMMEND AT LEAST 8 OZ. PER WEEK	
	Moderate to high in Omega-3 fatty acids, greater than or equal to 1 gram per 3.5 oz.	**Lower in Omega-3 fatty acids, less than 1 gram per 3.5 oz.**
Finfish (Cont'd)	Salmon, chum Salmon, coho Salmon, pink Salmon, sockeye Sardine, Atlantic Sardine, Pacific Saury Scad, Muroaji Sprat Sturgeon, Atlantic Trout, lake Tuna, albacore Tuna, bluefin Whitefish, lake	Flounder, Yellowtail Grouper, jewfish Grouper, red Haddock Hake, Atlantic Hake, Pacific Hake, red Hake, silver Hake, unspecified Halibut, Atlantic Halibut, Greenland Halibut, Pacific Mackerel, horse Mahi mahi Mullet, striped Ocean perch Orange roughy Perch, white Perch, yellow Pike, northern Pike, walleye Plaice, European Pollock Pompano, Florida Ratfish Rockfish, brown Rockfish, canary Rockfish, unspecified Scad, other

	Moderate to high in Omega-3 fatty acids, greater than or equal to 1 gram per 3.5 oz.	Lower in Omega-3 fatty acids, less than 1 gram per 3.5 oz.
Finfish (Cont'd)		Scrod
		Sea bass, Japanese
		Seatrout, sand
		Seatrout, spotted
		Shark
		Sheepshead
		Smelt, pond
		Smelt, rainbow
		Smelt, sweet
		Snapper, red
		Sole, European
		Spot
		Sturgeon, common
		Sunfish, pumpkinseed
		Swordfish
		Trout, arctic char
		Trout, brook
		Trout, rainbow
		Tuna, skipjack
		Tuna, unspecified
		Tuna, yellowfin
		Turbot
		Whiting, European
		Wolffish, Atlantic
Mollusks	Conch, unspecified	Abalone, New Zealand
		Abalone, South African
		Clam, hardshell
		Clam, hen
		Clam, Japanese hardshell

ACCEPTABLE — Recommend at least 8 oz. per week

	Moderate to high in Omega-3 fatty acids, greater than or equal to 1 gram per 3.5 oz.	Lower in Omega-3 fatty acids, less than 1 gram per 3.5 oz.
Mollusks (Cont'd)		Clam, littleneck
		Clam, softshell
		Clam, surf
		Cuttlefish, unspecified
		Mussel, blue
		Mussel, Mediterranean
		Octopus, common
		Oyster, eastern
		Oyster, European
		Oyster, Pacific
		Periwinkle, common
		Scallop, Atlantic deepsea
		Scallop, calico
		Scallop, unspecified
		Squid, Atlantic
		Squid, short-finned
		Squid, unspecified
		Whelk, unspecified

Poultry and Game

Lean, less than 1 gram fat per ounce
Poultry and game meats listed in this category are very lean and may be eaten as often as desired. Poultry products should be skinned and have all visible fat removed before cooking.

Medium fat, between 1-3 grams fat per ounce
These choices are higher in fat content but are still better choices than most red meats.

NOT RECOMMENDED

High fat, greater than 3 grams fat per ounce
Poultry and game with greater than 3 grams fat per ounce are not recommended.

NOTE

- Fresh poultry contains approximately 25-30 mg. sodium per ounce. Most poultry products do not usually provide nutrition labeling; therefore, sodium symbols are not used in this section.

BRAND	ACCEPTABLE		NOT RECOMMENDED
	Lean, less than 1 gram fat per oz.	Medium fat, between 1-3 grams fat per oz.	High fat, greater than 3 grams fat per oz.

Chicken	Broilers or fryers:
	  Breast
		Broilers or fryers:
		  Dark meat
		  Drumstick
		  Leg
		  Light meat
		  Wing
		Roasting:
		  Dark meat
		  Light meat
		Stewing:
		  Light meat
			All poultry with skin
			Broilers or fryers:
			  Back
			  Thigh
			Stewing:
			  Dark meat

Duck		Wild duck: Breast	Domesticated duck
Elk	Elk: All parts		
Goose			Domesticated goose
Guinea	Guinea		
Hare		Hare: All parts	
Opossum		Opossum: All parts	

Pheasant	Pheasant:
	  Breast
		Pheasant:
		  Leg	

Quail	Quail:
	  Breast
		Quail:
		  All other parts	

BRAND	ACCEPTABLE		NOT RECOMMENDED
	Lean, less than 1 gram fat per oz.	Medium fat, between 1-3 grams fat per oz.	High fat, greater than 3 grams ° fat per oz.
Rabbit		Rabbit: All parts	
Squab (pigeon)		Squab: All parts	

Turkey	Fryer-Roasters:
	 Breast
	 Light meat
	 Wing
	The Turkey Store™ Premium
	 Fresh Turkey:
	  100% ground breast meat
	Young toms:
	 Light meat
		Fryer-Roasters:
		 Back
		 Dark meat
		 Leg
		Mr. Turkey™ ground turkey
		The Turkey Store™ Premium
		 Fresh Turkey:
		  Lean ground
		Young hens:
		 Dark meat
		 Light meat
		Young toms:
		 Dark meat
		 Leg
			Louis Rich™ ground turkey
			Young toms:
			 Back
			 Wing

Venison	Venison: All parts		

Lunchmeats

Lunchmeats which have been specially processed to lower fat are acceptable in limited quantities.

■ **Contain 50% or less calories from fat (comparable to lean meat) (LIMIT USE)**

Products listed in this category are the leanest and are preferred choices. Remember that because of their high sodium and nitrite content, consumption of all lunchmeats should be limited.

■ **Contain 51% to 65% calories from fat (comparable to medium fat meat) (LIMIT USE)**

These lunchmeats are higher in fat but still acceptable in limited amounts. Use these choices less often.

NOT RECOMMENDED

■ **Contain greater than 65% of calories from fat**

Lunchmeats with greater than 65% of calories from fat are not recommended. Note that most turkey franks and bologna fall in this category.

NOTE

■ Most lunchmeats are high in sodium because they are processed with salt and sodium nitrites. Sodium nitrite is used as a preservative and high intake is associated with increased cancer risk. For these reasons, it is best to limit consumption of all processed lunchmeats. The average sodium content of most lunchmeat is between 300-400 mg. per one ounce serving. The sodium content of some lunchmeats, such as ham, can be reduced by rinsing the slice before using. Since this procedure rinses off much of the sodium preservative, you should only rinse off what you are going to use. Sodium symbols are used to indicate high (▲) or low (▽) sodium **only** when sodium content is provided on the product label. Those products that are not identified with either symbol may be either high or low sodium or contain between 141-399 mg. sodium per serving.

BRAND	ACCEPTABLE		NOT RECOMMENDED
	Contain 50% or less calories from fat (comparable to lean meat) (LIMIT USE)	Contain 51% to 65% calories from fat (comparable to medium fat meat) (LIMIT USE)	Contain greater than 65% of calories from fat
Armour	*Sliced dried beef*		*Turkey breakfast strips*
Best		*Lower fat Kosher bologna*	*Beef knacks* *Kosher bologna* Kosher corned beef Kosher franks *Kosher pastrami* Kosher salami Lower fat Kosher frankfurter Lower fat Kosher salami
Butterball	Chicken breast Chopped turkey ham Turkey breast (oven roasted) Turkey breast (smoked) Turkey ham Turkey pastrami	Turkey salami ▲Turkey smoked sausage	Bun size turkey franks Turkey bologna
Country Club	Corned beef Imported cooked ham Thin sliced smoked beef	Thin sliced ham Thin sliced smoked chicken Thin sliced smoked turkey	*Polish Kielbasa*
Ekrich	Cooked ham Honey style loaf Lean slender sliced turkey Lean sliced: Corned beef Sliced beef Smoked ham		Beef bologna Beef franks Beef smoky-links Beer salami Bologna Cotto beef salami Franks

▲ High sodium, 400 mg. or greater per serving.

BRAND	ACCEPTABLE		NOT RECOMMENDED
	Contain 50% or less calories from fat (comparable to lean meat) (LIMIT USE)	Contain 51% to 65% calories from fat (comparable to medium fat meat) (LIMIT USE)	Contain greater than 65% of calories from fat
Ekrich (Cont'd)	Lite cooked ham Lite lower salt ham ▲New England brand sausage		Garlic bologna Ham and cheese loaf Jumbo cheese franks *Lean Supreme bologna* *Lean Supreme franks* Lite bologna Lite franks Lite Polish kielbasa Lite Smok-Y-Links Old fashioned loaf Olive loaf Original smoky-links Pickle loaf Polish kielbasa Thin sliced bologna
Empire		Turkey Franks	
Hillshire Farms	Deli Select: ▽Corned Beef – 98% fat free ▽Honey Ham – 96% fat free ▽Honey roasted turkey breast 98% fat free ▽Oven roasted turkey breast 98% fat free ▽Pastrami – 98% fat free ▽Smoked beef – 98% fat free		

▲ High sodium, 400 mg. or greater per serving.
▽ Low sodium, 140 mg. or less per serving.

BRAND	ACCEPTABLE		NOT RECOMMENDED
	Contain 50% or less calories from fat (comparable to lean meat) (LIMIT USE)	Contain 51% to 65% calories from fat (comparable to medium fat meat) (LIMIT USE)	Contain greater than 65% of calories from fat
Hillshire Farms (Cont'd)	Deli Select (Cont'd): ▽Smoked chicken breast 98% fat free ▽Smoked turkey breast 98% fat free ▽Turkey Ham – 96% fat free		
Holly Farms			Cheese chicken franks Chicken bologna Chicken franks
Hormel		Light and Lean: ▲90% fat free franks	
HyGrade			Ball Park Franks Beef bologna Beef franks Bologna Grill Master: Chicken bologna Chicken cheese franks Chicken franks Turkey franks Lite Ball Park Franks Salami
Louis Rich	Honey roasted turkey breast Oven roasted deluxe chicken breast	Oven roasted white chicken Turkey pastrami	Cheese turkey franks Turkey Bologna (82% fat free) Turkey cotto salami

▲ High sodium, 400 mg. or greater per serving.
▽ Low sodium, 140 mg. or less per serving.

BRAND	ACCEPTABLE		NOT RECOMMENDED
	Contain 50% or less calories from fat (comparable to lean meat) (LIMIT USE)	Contain 51% to 65% calories from fat (comparable to medium fat meat) (LIMIT USE)	Contain greater than 65% of calories from fat
Louis Rich (Cont'd)	Sliced deli-thin: Hickory smoked turkey breast 98% fat free ▽Oven roasted chicken breast 96% fat free Oven roasted turkey breast 97% fat free Smoked turkey ham 96% fat free Turkey pastrami – 96% fat free Smoked turkey – 96% fat free Turkey ham Turkey smoked sausage 90% fat free		Turkey franks Turkey salami
Morning Star Farms		▲Breakfast patties Grillers	Breakfast links (cholesterol free) Breakfast strips
Mr. Turkey	Smoked turkey ham Turkey breast	Turkey cotto salami	Cheese franks Turkey bologna Turkey franks
Oscar Meyer	Baked cooked ham Boiled ham Honey ham Honey loaf Lower salt ham Smoked cooked ham		Beef bologna Beef franks (bun length) Bologna Braunschweiger Cheese hot dogs Cotto salami

▲ High sodium, 400 mg. or greater per serving.
▽ Low sodium, 140 mg. or less per serving.

BRAND	ACCEPTABLE		NOT RECOMMENDED
	Contain 50% or less calories from fat (comparable to lean meat) (LIMIT USE)	Contain 51% to 65% calories from fat (comparable to medium fat meat) (LIMIT USE)	Contain greater than 65% of calories from fat
Oscar Meyer (Cont'd)			*Ham and cheese* Hard salami Liver cheese *New England brand sausage* Salami for beer Wieners
Rath Black Hawk			Hot dogs made with chicken pork and beef
The Turkey Store			Breakfast sausage
Thornapple Valley			Braunschweiger Liverwurst Polish kielbasa sausage Red Hot Franks Smoked sausage

PREPARED MIXES

This section contains listings for the following food categories:

◇ Baking Mixes
◇ Batter and Coating Mixes
◇ Pudding and Gelatin Mixes

These products offer convenience and variety but at the same time can be very high in calories from fat and simple sugar. They may also contain substantial amounts of sodium. Use these food products sparingly. Some products such as low calorie gelatin and pudding are low in fat and simple sugar and can therefore be used more often.

Baking Mixes

ACCEPTABLE

■ **Without added fat (LIMIT USE)**
Baking mixes in this category are preferred because they are processed without added fat. This allows you to add acceptable oil (try reducing the amount of oil by at least half) and other ingredients such as egg whites and skim milk at home when you are preparing the food item. Many of these products are high in simple sugar.

■ **With added unsaturated fat (LIMIT USE),** and

■ **With added acceptable partially hydrogenated oil or shortening (LIMIT USE)**
This and the preceding category contain baking mixes with added acceptable fats.

NOT RECOMMENDED

■ **With added saturated fat**
Baking mixes with added saturated fat are not recommended.

NOTE

■ Sodium content of processed baking mixes is variable depending on the type of product and can range between 40-600 mg. per serving. Sodium symbols are used to indicate high (▲) or low (▽) sodium **only** when sodium content is provided on the product label. Those products that are not identified with either symbol may be either high or low sodium or contain between 141-399 mg. sodium per serving.

BRAND	ACCEPTABLE			NOT RECOMMENDED
	Without added fat (LIMIT USE)	With added unsaturated fat (LIMIT USE)	With added acceptable partially hydrogenated oil or shortening (LIMIT USE)	With added saturated fat
Arrowhead Mills	★Bran muffin mixes *Cornbread mix* *Griddle lite pancake mix* ★Oatbran pancake and waffle mix ▲★Pancake and waffle mix			Biscuit mix
Aunt Jemima	▲Original pancake mix ▲★Whole wheat pancake and waffle mix with oatbran		▲•Buttermilk complete pancake & waffle mix ▲•Complete pancake & waffle mix ▲★•Lite buttermilk complete pancake mix Pancake express mix: ▲•Buttermilk	

Betty Crocker	Angel food cake mix		▲Bisquick variety baking and pancake mix
			Brownie mix:
			  ▽Frosted
			  ▽Fudge
			Creamy deluxe frosting:
			  ▽Amaretto almond
			  ▽Cherry
				Brownie mix:
				  Bakeshop chunky chocolate walnut
				  Chocolate chip
				  German chocolate
				  Classics date bar mix
				Creamy deluxe frosting:
				  Chocolate chip
				  Coconut pecan

▲ High sodium, 400 mg. or greater per serving.
▽ Low sodium, 140 mg. or less per serving.
★ High fiber, 3 g. or greater per serving.
• Contains egg yolks.

BRAND	ACCEPTABLE			NOT RECOMMENDED
	Without added fat (LIMIT USE)	With added unsaturated fat (LIMIT USE)	With added acceptable partially hydrogenated oil or shortening (LIMIT USE)	With added saturated fat
Betty Crocker (Cont'd)			Creamy deluxe frosting (Cont'd): ▽Chocolate ▽Cream cheese ▽Vanilla Creamy deluxe party frosting: ▽Chocolate with dinosaurs ▽Vanilla with teddy bears Devils food cake mix with chocolate frosting Frosting mix: ▽Chocolate fudge Gingerbread cake and cookie mix MicroRave: Brownies Yellow cake mix with chocolate frosting Muffin mix: ▽Blueberry Carrot nut Cinnamon streusel Oat bran Strawberry crown	Creamy deluxe frosting (Cont'd): Rainbow chip Creamy deluxe party frosting: Chocolate with chocolate chips Frosting mix: Coconut pecan *Vanilla* MicroRave: German chocolate cake with coconut pecan frosting Muffin mix: *Bakeshop blueberry* *Bakeshop Dutch apple* *Chocolate chip* Oatmeal raisin Pineapple upside down cake Supermoist cake mix: Chocolate chip Rainbow chip Supermoist cake mix, pudding in the mix: Chocolate chip Chocolate chocolate chip

▽ Low sodium, 140 mg. or less per serving.

BRAND	ACCEPTABLE			NOT RECOMMENDED
	Without added fat (LIMIT USE)	With added unsaturated fat (LIMIT USE)	With added acceptable partially hydrogenated oil or shortening (LIMIT USE)	With added saturated fat

Betty Crocker (Cont'd)			▽Pie crust mix
			Pie crust sticks
			Pound cake mix
			Supermoist cake mix:
			  Butter recipe chocolate
			  Cherry chip
			  ▲Chocolate fudge
			  ▲Devil's food
			  White cake
			  Yellow cake
			Supermoist cake mix, pudding in the mix:
			  Carrot cake
			  German chocolate
			  Golden vanilla
				Supreme brownie mix:
				  Caramel brownies

Bisquick			▲Baking mix
			Shake 'n pour:
			  ▲•Apple-cinnamon pancake mix
			  ▲•Blueberry pancake mix
			  ▲•Buttermilk pancake mix	

Cafe du Monde				Beignet mix: French doughnuts

▲ High sodium, 400 mg. or greater per serving.
▽ Low sodium, 140 mg. or less per serving.
• Contains egg yolks.

BRAND	ACCEPTABLE			NOT RECOMMENDED
	Without added fat (LIMIT USE)	With added unsaturated fat (LIMIT USE)	With added acceptable partially hydrogenated oil or shortening (LIMIT USE)	With added saturated fat
Classique Fare				Belgian waffle mix Pancake mix: Apple

Duncan Hines			Bakery style muffin mix:
			  Blueberry with crumb
			    topping
			  Cinnamon swirl
			Brownie mix:
			  ▽Chewy fudge
			  ▽Double fudge
			  ▽Milk chocolate
			Cake mix:
			  Butter recipe golden
			  Devil's food
			  Fudge marble
			  Lemon supreme
			  Yellow
			▽Dutch Fudge Frosting
			Layer Cake ready-to-
			  spread frostings:
			    ▽Chocolate
			    ▽Vanilla
			Muffin mix:
			  Oatbran blueberry
			  Oatbran honey
			  Wild blueberry
				Brownie mix:
				  Peanut butter fudge
				  Turtle
				Chocolate chip cookie mix
				Home recipe peanut butter
				  cookie mix
				Tiara dessert kits:
				  All flavors
				Triple fudge truffle

▽ Low sodium, 140 mg. or less per serving.

BRAND	ACCEPTABLE			NOT RECOMMENDED
	Without added fat (LIMIT USE)	With added unsaturated fat (LIMIT USE)	With added acceptable partially hydrogenated oil or shortening (LIMIT USE)	With added saturated fat
Duncan Hines (Cont'd)			Sheetcake frosting: ▽Chocolate ▽Vanilla	

Estee	▽Pancake mix		▽Brownie mix
			Cake mix:
			  ▽Chocolate
			  ▽Lemon
			  ▽Pound
			  ▽White	

Fast Shake			Blueberry pancake mix Buttermilk pancake mix	
Fearn				Bran muffin mix Carob cake mix Carrot cake mix Spice cake mix
Featherweight		▽Complete pancake mix		
Golden Dipt	•Funnel cake mix			
Golden Harvest	Muffin mix: ▽★•Oat bran			
Hain	▲★Whole wheat baking mix			

▲ High sodium, 400 mg. or greater per serving.
▽ Low sodium, 140 mg. or less per serving.
★ High fiber, 3 g. or greater per serving.
• Contains egg yolks.

BRAND	ACCEPTABLE			NOT RECOMMENDED
	Without added fat (LIMIT USE)	With added unsaturated fat (LIMIT USE)	With added acceptable partially hydrogenated oil or shortening (LIMIT USE)	With added saturated fat
Hodgson Mills	Corn meal mix	▽Buckwheat pancake mix Buttermilk pancake mix Cornbread *Insta-bake baking mix* Muffin mix: Bran Whole wheat		Gingerbread
Hungry Jack	Pancake mix: ▲Original extra-light		Pancake mix: ▲•Buttermilk	
Jiffy			Baking mix	Brownie mix Buttermilk biscuit mix Cake mixes: All flavors Cornbread mix Frosting mix: Fudge White Muffin mixes: All flavors Pie crust mix
Kroger			▽Brownie mix Muffin mix: Corn bran	*Complete pancake mix* Extra Moist cake mix: All flavors

▲ High sodium, 400 mg. or greater per serving.
▽ Low sodium, 140 mg. or less per serving.
• Contains egg yolks.

BRAND	ACCEPTABLE			NOT RECOMMENDED
	Without added fat (LIMIT USE)	With added unsaturated fat (LIMIT USE)	With added acceptable partially hydrogenated oil or shortening (LIMIT USE)	With added saturated fat
Kroger (Cont'd)			Muffin mix (Cont'd): Oat bran Rice bran Pancake and waffle mix: ▲•Buttermilk	Frosting: Creamy fudge Creamy white *Graham cracker crumbs*
Martha White			Muffin mix: Double blueberry	Brownie mix: Double fudge chunk Corn muffin mix
Mrs. Butterworth's	▲Old fashioned pancake mix		▲•Buttermilk complete pancake mix ▲•Complete pancake mix	
Nabisco				Graham cracker crumbs
Nature's Best				White cake mix
Pillsbury	Frost It Hot frosting mix: ▽Fluffy white ▽Whipped chocolate flavored Hot roll mix Lovin' Lites: Blueberry muffin mix Chocolate fudge frosting Devil's food cake mix		Bread mix: Banana *Date* Nut Fudge Brownie mix: ▽Microwave Bundt cake: *Boston creme*	Brownie mix: *Deluxe fudge* Frosting supreme: Chocolate chip Coconut pecan Pillsbury plus cake mix: Chocolate chip cookie

▲ High sodium, 400 mg. or greater per serving.
▽ Low sodium, 140 mg. or less per serving.
• Contains egg yolks.

Brand	Acceptable			Not Recommended
	Without added fat (LIMIT USE)	**With added unsaturated fat (LIMIT USE)**	**With added acceptable partially hydrogenated oil or shortening (LIMIT USE)**	**With added saturated fat**

Pillsbury (Cont'd)	Lovin' Lites (Cont'd):
	    Fudge brownie mix
	    Vanilla frosting
	    Yellow cake mix
	Lovin' Loaf:
	    Angel food cake mix
			Bundt cake (Cont'd):
			    Pineapple cream cake
			        mix
			Frosting supreme:
			    ▽Chocolate fudge
			    ▽Lemon
			    ▽Milk chocolate
			    ▽Vanilla flavor
			Funfetti frosting:
			    ▽Pink vanilla flavor
			Great Additions brownie
			    mix:
			        ▽Walnut
			Microwave cake and
			    frosting mix
			Pillsbury plus cake mix:
			    Banana
			    Dark chocolate
			    Devil's food
			    Funfetti
			    German chocolate
			    Lemon
			    White
			    Yellow
			    Streusel swirl	

Spruance				*Bread mix*
Swans Down	Cake flour			

▽ Low sodium, 140 mg. or less per serving.

BRAND	ACCEPTABLE			NOT RECOMMENDED
	Without added fat (LIMIT USE)	With added unsaturated fat (LIMIT USE)	With added acceptable partially hydrogenated oil or shortening (LIMIT USE)	With added saturated fat
Sweet 'n Low			Cake mix: ▽All flavors Frosting mix: ▽White ▽Pancake mix	
Uncle Ben's	Rite bran: ▽Pure rice bran			
Ye Olde Tyme			Cobbler crust mix •Sopaipilla mix	

▽ Low sodium, 140 mg. or less per serving.
• Contains egg yolks.

Batter and Coating Mixes

■ **Without added fat**
These mixes are preferred because they do not contain added fat. We do **not** recommend using these mixes for deep fat frying. A more healthful alternative is to use these mixes to coat meat or poultry then bake in a hot oven (400-450°) with only enough oil to lightly coat the baking pan. Turn meat halfway through the baking time for a crispy texture.

■ **With added unsaturated fat,** and

■ **With added acceptable partially hydrogenated oil or shortening**
This and the preceding category contain mixes with added acceptable fat.

NOT RECOMMENDED

■ **With added saturated fat or batter mix designed only for deep fat frying**
Mixes with added saturated fat or batter mixes designed only for deep fat frying are not recommended.

NOTE

■ Coating mixes contain variable amounts of sodium and can range from 200-800 mg. per serving. Sodium symbols are used to indicate high (▲) or low (▽) sodium **only** when sodium content is provided on the product label. Those products that are not identified with either symbol may be either high or low sodium or contain between 141-399 mg. sodium per serving.

BRAND	ACCEPTABLE			NOT RECOMMENDED
	Without added fat	With added unsaturated fat	With added acceptable partially hydrogenated oil or shortening	With added saturated fat or batter mix designed only for deep fat frying
Don's Chuck Wagon Kitchen				All purpose onion ring mix Batter mix *Chiles rellenos batter mix* Golden mushroom batter mix
Drakes				Crispy fry mix
Fantastic Foods				Tempura batter mix
Fry Krisp	•Country style coating for steaks and chops •Cracker meal •Old fashioned seafood mix		•Krispy country chicken mix	Batter mix Onion ring mix
Fryin' Magic	Coating mix			

Golden Dipt	Chicken frying mix
	Seasoned frying mix:
	  Fish fry
	  Seafood
		All purpose breading
		All purpose cracker meal
		Cracker meal
				All purpose batter mix
				Batter mix:
				  English style fish and chips
				  Tempura
				Cornmeal mix with onion:
				  Hush puppy
				Corny dog batter mix
				Donut batter mix
				Hush puppy mix
				Japanese style tempura batter mix (no salt added)

Kellogg's	Corn flake crumbs			

• Contains egg yolks.

BRAND	ACCEPTABLE			NOT RECOMMENDED
	Without added fat	With added unsaturated fat	With added acceptable partially hydrogenated oil or shortening	With added saturated fat or batter mix designed only for deep fat frying
Kentucky Kernal	Seasoned flour			
Kroger				Cracker meal
Nabisco	▽Cracker meal			
Nona Bella's				Genuine golden fish fry breading
Shake 'n Bake			▲Bar-B-Q flavor coating ▲Coating for chicken *Coating for fish* Coating for pork ▲Oven fry extra-crispy chicken coating ▲Oven fry crispy for pork ▲Oven fry homestyle chicken	

▲ High sodium, 400 mg. or greater per serving.
▽ Low sodium, 140 mg. or less per serving.

Pudding and Gelatin Mixes

■ Without added fat

These mixes are preferred because they do not have added fat. Remember that some of these selections may contain large amounts of refined sugar. You may choose to select those items that are low calorie or sugar free. For a discussion on use of artificial sweeteners see pg. 31. Puddings should be made with skim milk.

With added acceptable unsaturated oil

Our product survey revealed that there were no products fitting this criteria.

With added acceptable partially hydrogenated oil or shortening

These mixes have added acceptable fats.

NOT RECOMMENDED

■ With added saturated fat

Pudding and gelatin mixes with added saturated fat are not recommended.

NOTE

- The sodium content of pudding is approximately 110-140 mg. per ½ cup serving. Most gelatins contain approximately 50-70 mg. sodium per ½ cup serving. Sodium symbols are used to indicate high (▲) or low (▽) sodium **only** when sodium content is provided on the product label. Those products that are not identified with either symbol may be either high or low sodium or contain between 141-399 mg. sodium per serving.

Brand	Acceptable			Not Recommended
	Without added fat	**With added acceptable unsaturated oil**	**With added partially hydrogenated oil or shortening**	**With added saturated fat**
Bascom's	Tapioca			
D-Zerta				Whipped topping mix
Del Monte			Pudding cups: All flavors	
Dia Mel	Gel-A-Thin: ▽*All flavors*			
Dream Whip				Whipped topping mix
Estee	▽*Low calorie cherry gelatin* Reduced calorie instant pudding and pie filling: ▽*Chocolate* ▽*Vanilla*			Whipped topping mix
General Foods	Minute tapioca			
Hunt's			▽Snack pack ▽Snack pack light	
International Bazaar				Mousse instant dessert mix: All flavors
Jell-O	Microwave pudding and pie filling: ▽All flavors (except milk chocolate)		Instant pudding: All flavors (except milk chocolate)	1-2-3 Gelatin with two toppings Americana tapioca pudding

▽ Low sodium, 140 mg. or less per serving.

BRAND	ACCEPTABLE			NOT RECOMMENDED
	Without added fat	With added acceptable unsaturated oil	With added partially hydrogenated oil or shortening	With added saturated fat
Jell-O (Cont'd)	Pudding and pie filling: ▽All flavors (except lemon) Regular gelatin: ▽All flavors Sugar free gelatin: ▽All flavors Sugar free instant pudding: All flavors Sugar free pudding and pie filling: ▽All flavors			Cheesecake: New York style Real Chocolate mousse pie Instant pudding: Milk chocolate Microwave pudding and pie filling: Milk chocolate No Bake: Coconut cream pie Pie mix: Chocolate mousse Coconut cream *Pumpkin* Pudding and pie filling: Lemon
Knox	▽Unflavored gelatin			
Kroger	•Egg custard mix Instant pudding: All flavors (except chocolate chip) Pudding & pie filling: All flavors (except coconut cream)			*Chocolate almond pudding* *Double chocolate pudding* Instant pudding: Chocolate chip *Mousse mix* Pudding & pie filling: Coconut cream

▽ Low sodium, 140 mg. or less per serving.
• Contains egg yolks.

BRAND	ACCEPTABLE			NOT RECOMMENDED
	Without added fat	**With added acceptable unsaturated oil**	**With added partially hydrogenated oil or shortening**	**With added saturated fat**
Kroger (Cont'd)	Regular gelatins: All flavors Sugar free gelatins: ▽All flavors Sugar free pudding: All flavors (except pistachio)			Select chocolate dessert mix: Chocolate almond Double chocolate Sugar free pudding: Pistachio Whipped topping mix
Nabisco Royal				*Cheesecake mix
Salada	Junket Danish Dessert pie glaze filling			Ice cream mix: *All flavors
Sans Sucre				Cheesecake mousse Sugar free chocolate mousse
Sweet 'n Low	Pudding mix: *Lemon* *Vanilla*		Custard mixes: ▽All flavors	
Thank You			Smooth 'n creamy pudding: All flavors	
Weight Watchers	Instant pudding: Chocolate ▲Vanilla			Lite whip mousse Mousse dessert mix: All flavors

▲ High sodium, 400 mg. or greater per serving.
▽ Low sodium, 140 mg. or less per serving.
* This product contains acceptable ingredients, however, the recipe requires the addition of ingredients that are high in total and saturated fat.

SNACK FOODS

This section contains listings for the following food categories:

◇ Chips, Pretzels and Other Snacks
◇ Cookies and Fruit Bars
◇ Crackers
◇ Popcorn (Ready Made)
◇ Popping Corn (Plain or Microwave)

These products add variety to the diet. Unfortunately if quantities are not carefully controlled they can also contribute to excessive calories from fat and simple sugar. Over time, these excesses can translate to unwanted weight gain. Most snack foods are also high in sodium.

Chips, Pretzels and Other Snacks

ACCEPTABLE

■ **Without added fat and/or lowfat, 2 grams fat or less per 1 ounce serving (may be partially hydrogenated), may be high in sodium**
These are preferable choices because they are low in fat and therefore low in calories.

■ **With added unsaturated oil, most are high in fat and sodium (LIMIT USE), and**

■ **With added acceptable partially hydrogenated oil or shortening, most are high in fat and sodium (LIMIT USE)**
Snack foods listed in this and the preceding category contain added acceptable fats but most are high in fat and therefore high in calories. Limited use is recommended.

NOT RECOMMENDED

■ **With added saturated fat**
Snacks with added saturated fat are not recommended.

NOTE

■ Most snack foods are high in sodium. For example, potato chips contain approximately 150-400 mg. sodium per 1 ounce serving. Sodium symbols are used to indicate high (▲) or low (▽) sodium **only** when sodium content is provided on the product label. Those products that are not identified with either symbol may be either high or low sodium or contain between 141-399 mg. sodium per serving.

BRAND	ACCEPTABLE			NOT RECOMMENDED
	Without added fat and/or lowfat, 2 grams fat or less per 1 ounce serving (may be partially hydrogenated) may be high in sodium	With added unsaturated oil most are high in fat and sodium (LIMIT USE)	With added acceptable partially hydrogenated oil or shortening most are high in fat and sodium (LIMIT USE)	With added saturated fat

Angonoa's			Breadsticks:
			  Garlic
			  Italian
			  ▽Low Sodium
			  Sesame royale
			Mini breadsticks:
			  Sesame
			  Whole wheat with sesame
				Breadsticks:
				  Cheese
				Mini breadsticks:
				  Cheese-sesame

Arrowhead Mills	Blue corn curls: ▽★Unsalted	▽★Unsalted blue corn chips		

Barbara's	100% whole wheat sunflower snack sticks
	▽Crackle snax
	Oat bran pretzels – unsalted:
	  ▽Whole wheat flour plus >25% pure oat bran
	  Whole wheat flour plus >30% oat bran
		100% whole wheat pretzels with sesame seeds:
		  ▽No salt added
		  Regular (large)
		  Regular (small)
		100% whole wheat sesame sticks
		Bagel chips:
		  100% whole wheat
		Blue corn chips
		Natural potato chips
		Pinto chips (regular)
		▽Unsalted potato chips
				Cheese puff lights
				Natural cheese puffs
				Pinto chips with nacho cheese

▽ Low sodium, 140 mg. or less per serving.
★ High fiber, 3 g. or greater per serving.

BRAND	ACCEPTABLE			NOT RECOMMENDED
	Without added fat and/or lowfat, 2 grams fat or less per 1 ounce serving (may be partially hydrogenated) may be high in sodium	With added unsaturated oil most are high in fat and sodium (LIMIT USE)	With added acceptable partially hydrogenated oil or shortening most are high in fat and sodium (LIMIT USE)	With added saturated fat
Barney's		Crunchy potato chips		
Big Value			Corn chips ▲Party pretzels ▲Thin twist pretzels	Cheese puffs
Burns and Ricker			Bagel chips: 　All flavors Bagel crisps	
Butterfield			French fried crisp potato sticks Potato sticks	
Cabana			Potato chips	
Cain's (Snack Time)			Potato chips: 　Bar-B-Q 　Marcelle dip style 　▽Marcelle dip style, no salt added 　▲Salt and vinegar 　Thin	Potato chips: 　Sour cream and onion
Camacho		Nacho corn chips		Tortilla corn chips: 　Chili and cheese

▲ High sodium, 400 mg. or greater per serving.
▽ Low sodium, 140 mg. or less per serving.

BRAND	ACCEPTABLE			NOT RECOMMENDED
	Without added fat and/or lowfat, 2 grams fat or less per 1 ounce serving (may be partially hydrogenated) may be high in sodium	With added unsaturated oil most are high in fat and sodium (LIMIT USE)	With added acceptable partially hydrogenated oil or shortening most are high in fat and sodium (LIMIT USE)	With added saturated fat
Cape Cod		Potato chips: ▽No salt added Party size ▽Regular		
Cheese Shop/Deli			Nacho chips: ▽No salt added ▽Plain Tortilla chips: ▽Traditional	Nacho chips: Cheese flavor
Chi Chi's			Tortilla chips: Plain	
Chico San	Mini rice cakes: ▽All flavors Popcorn cakes: ▽All flavors Rice cakes: ▽All flavors			
Combos				Crackers with cheddar cheese *Crackers with peanut butter filling* Filled pretzels: Cheddar cheese filling Cheese pizza Nacho cheese

▽ Low sodium, 140 mg. or less per serving.

BRAND	ACCEPTABLE			NOT RECOMMENDED
	Without added fat and/or lowfat, 2 grams fat or less per 1 ounce serving (may be partially hydrogenated) may be high in sodium	With added unsaturated oil most are high in fat and sodium (LIMIT USE)	With added acceptable partially hydrogenated oil or shortening most are high in fat and sodium (LIMIT USE)	With added saturated fat

Cornnuts			Toasted corn:
			  Barbecue
			  Original
				Toasted corn:
				  Nacho cheese

Country Oven			*Potato chips*	

Delta Gold			Potato chips:
			  Dip style
			  Regular	

Dos Hombres			▽Authentic blue chips	

Eagle	▲Bavarian hard pretzels	Hawaiian Kettle extra crunchy potato chips:
		  Regular
		Potato chips:
		  Idaho russet, dark and crunchy
		  Ridges
		  Thins
			Hawaiian Kettle extra crunchy potato chips:
			  Barbecue
			Potato chips:
			  Extra crunchy Louisiana BBQ
			  Mesquite barbecue thins
				All natural pretzels
				Cheese crunch
				Potato chips:
				  Ranch (ridged)
				  Ridged, sour cream and onion
				Snack mix
				Tortilla chips:
				  Nacho cheese
				  Ranch

Estee	▽Sodium free unsalted pretzels			
Featherweight			▽Unsalted potato chips	Low sodium cheese curls Low sodium corn chips

▲ High sodium, 400 mg. or greater per serving.
▽ Low sodium, 140 mg. or less per serving.

BRAND	ACCEPTABLE			NOT RECOMMENDED
	Without added fat and/or lowfat, 2 grams fat or less per 1 ounce serving (may be partially hydrogenated) may be high in sodium	With added unsaturated oil most are high in fat and sodium (LIMIT USE)	With added acceptable partially hydrogenated oil or shortening most are high in fat and sodium (LIMIT USE)	With added saturated fat
Featherweight (Cont'd)				*Low sodium nacho tortillas* *Low sodium round tortilla chips*
Flavor House				*Party mix*
Flavor Tree			▽No salt party mix ▽No salt sesame sticks Sesame chips Sesame sticks	Party mix: 　Hot 'n Spicey Party mix with sesame sticks Sesame sticks: 　Cheddar cheese 　Sour cream and onion
Frito Lay		Crunch tators: 　▽Mighty mesquite 　▽Original	Doritos: 　▽Toasted corn lightly salted Fritos: 　Bar-B-Q 　Crisp 'n Thin 　Dip size 　Original Funyons Munchos Potato chips: 　Bar-B-Q 　Regular	Chee-tos: 　Crunchy 　No cholesterol puffs Chee-tos light: 　Crunchy Doritos: 　Cool ranch 　Jumpin' Jack cheese 　Nacho cheese 　Salsa Rio flavor Doritos light: 　Cool ranch 　Nacho cheese

▽ Low sodium, 140 mg. or less per serving.

BRAND	ACCEPTABLE			NOT RECOMMENDED
	Without added fat and/or lowfat, 2 grams fat or less per 1 ounce serving (may be partially hydrogenated) may be high in sodium	With added unsaturated oil most are high in fat and sodium (LIMIT USE)	With added acceptable partially hydrogenated oil or shortening most are high in fat and sodium (LIMIT USE)	With added saturated fat
Frito Lay (Cont'd)			Potato chips (Cont'd): ▲Salt and vinegar Santitas: ▽Cantina style Tortilla chips Tortilla strips Tostitos: Traditional	Fritos: Chili cheese Wild n' Mild ranch Potato chips: *Cheddar cheese* Cheddar cheese and sour cream Sour cream and onion Tostitos: *Sharp nacho cheese*
General Mills				Bugles: Nacho cheese Regular
Guiltless Gourmet	No oil tortilla chips: ▽salted ▽unsalted			
Hain	Mini rice cakes: ▽Apple-cinnamon ▽Honey nut ▽Plain ▽Teriyaki	Mini rice cakes: ▽Barbecue Sesame tortilla chips Whole grain carrot chips		*Cheese sesame tortilla chips* Mini rice cakes: Cheese Taco style tortilla chips
Health Valley		Corn chips: ▽Crisp 'n Natural ▽*Natural potato chips*		Cheddar Lites: Cheddar cheese and green onion

▲ High sodium, 400 mg. or greater per serving.
▽ Low sodium, 140 mg. or less per serving.

BRAND	ACCEPTABLE			NOT RECOMMENDED
	Without added fat and/or lowfat, 2 grams fat or less per 1 ounce serving (may be partially hydrogenated) may be high in sodium	With added unsaturated oil most are high in fat and sodium (LIMIT USE)	With added acceptable partially hydrogenated oil or shortening most are high in fat and sodium (LIMIT USE)	With added saturated fat
Health Valley				Cheddar Lites (Cont'd): Original Corn chips: *with cheese*
Jay's		Jay's potato chips: *Barbecue* *Hotstuff* ▽*No salt added* ▽*Regular*		
Keebler	▲Butter pretzel braids ▲Butter pretzel knots ▲Butter pretzel nibblers		O'Boisies: Original Ripplin's: Barbecue Original Suncheros: Salsa Tato Skins: Barbecue *Regular*	Hooplahs crunch corn chips: Nacho flavor O'Boisies: Sour cream and onion Pizzarias: Cheese Zesty pepperoni Pop delux: Honey caramel glaze Ripplin's: Ranch Suncheros: Nacho Ranch

▲ High sodium, 400 mg. or greater per serving.
▽ Low sodium, 140 mg. or less per serving.

BRAND	ACCEPTABLE			NOT RECOMMENDED
	Without added fat and/or lowfat, 2 grams fat or less per 1 ounce serving (may be partially hydrogenated) may be high in sodium	With added unsaturated oil most are high in fat and sodium (LIMIT USE)	With added acceptable partially hydrogenated oil or shortening most are high in fat and sodium (LIMIT USE)	With added saturated fat
Keebler (Cont'd)				Tato Skins: Cheese n' Bacon Sour cream n' chives
Konricko	Rice cakes: ▽All flavors			
Kroger	Pretzels: ▲Bavarian style Oat bran ▲Rods ▲Sticks ▲Tiny thins ▲Twists		Corn chips: Bar-B-Q Regular Delicatessen Bagel chips: ▽All flavors Potato chips: Crisp and delicious Dip style *Sesame sticks* Tortilla chips: ▽Low salt restaurant style ▽Restaurant style ▽Traditional	Carmel corn and peanuts Cheese snax: Crunchy curls Puffed balls Pork rinds Tortilla chips: Nacho cheese
Krunchers		Potato chips: Jalapeño Mesquite Bar-B-Que Original		Potato chips: Alfredo

▲ High sodium, 400 mg. or greater per serving.
▽ Low sodium, 140 mg. or less per serving.

BRAND	ACCEPTABLE			NOT RECOMMENDED
	Without added fat and/or lowfat, 2 grams fat or less per 1 ounce serving (may be partially hydrogenated) may be high in sodium	With added unsaturated oil most are high in fat and sodium (LIMIT USE)	With added acceptable partially hydrogenated oil or shortening most are high in fat and sodium (LIMIT USE)	With added saturated fat
Lawry's			Cajun hot sticks *Honey roasted sesame sticks*	Jalapeño and cheddar flavor snack sticks Oat bran snack sticks
Lite Munchies		▽Barbecue ▽Toasted onion		Nacho cheese Rich chocolate
Little Bear Organic Foods		Bearitos: Blue corn tortilla chips – no salt Organic blue corn Bearitos tortilla chips: Original		Bearitos tortilla chips: Nacho flavored
Michael Seasons		Oat bran puffs: ▽Country spice ▽Original Oat bran tortillas: Lightly salted Salsa Potato chips: ▽Barbecue ▽Lightly salted ▽Unsalted ▽Wave cut dip chips		Potato chips: *Alfredo* Yogurt and green onion
Mother's	Rice cakes: ▽Corn ▽Multi-grain			

▽ Low sodium, 140 mg. or less per serving.

BRAND	ACCEPTABLE			NOT RECOMMENDED
	Without added fat and/or lowfat, 2 grams fat or less per 1 ounce serving (may be partially hydrogenated) may be high in sodium	With added unsaturated oil most are high in fat and sodium (LIMIT USE)	With added acceptable partially hydrogenated oil or shortening most are high in fat and sodium (LIMIT USE)	With added saturated fat
Mother's (Cont'd)	Rice cakes (Cont'd): ▽Plain ▽Sesame			
Nabisco	Mister Salty: ▲Dutch Pretzels ▲Sticks ▲Twists			Doo dads snack mix Mister Salty: Juniors
New York Style			Pita chips: *Garlic* *Hot 'n Spicey* *Onion* ▽*Plain, low sodium* *Rye with caraway*	
O'Grady				*Au gratin potato chips*
Pacific Rice	Crispy cakes: ▽Apple cinnamon ▽Italian spices ▽Natural ▽Natural-sodium free ▽Raisins 'n spice Mini crispys: ▽Apple spice ▽BBQ ▽Honey almond			Crispy cakes: Chili 'n cheese

▲ High sodium, 400 mg. or greater per serving.
▽ Low sodium, 140 mg. or less per serving.

BRAND	ACCEPTABLE			NOT RECOMMENDED
	Without added fat and/or lowfat, 2 grams fat or less per 1 ounce serving (may be partially hydrogenated) may be high in sodium	With added unsaturated oil most are high in fat and sodium (LIMIT USE)	With added acceptable partially hydrogenated oil or shortening most are high in fat and sodium (LIMIT USE)	With added saturated fat
Pacific Rice (Cont'd)	Mini crispys (Cont'd): ▽Honey sesame ▽Teriyaki			
Pepperidge Farm			Snack sticks: ▲Pretzel Pumpernickel Sesame	Snack mix: Classic Smoked Spicy Snack sticks: Three cheese
Planters		Corn chips	Bite-size tortilla chips: Traditional	Bite-size tortilla chips: Nacho cheese Cheez balls Cheez curls
Pringles		Corn Crisps: Corn flavor Idaho rippled: Mesquite BBQ Regular Potato chips: Regular Pringles light: ▽Regular		Corn Crisps: Tangy cheese flavor Idaho rippled: Cheddar cheese and sour cream French onion Potato chips: Cheez Ums Sour cream 'n onion Pringles light: Ranch

▲ High sodium, 400 mg. or greater per serving.
▽ Low sodium, 140 mg. or less per serving.

BRAND	ACCEPTABLE			NOT RECOMMENDED
	Without added fat and/or lowfat, 2 grams fat or less per 1 ounce serving (may be partially hydrogenated) may be high in sodium	With added unsaturated oil most are high in fat and sodium (LIMIT USE)	With added acceptable partially hydrogenated oil or shortening most are high in fat and sodium (LIMIT USE)	With added saturated fat
Pritikin	Rice cakes: ▽Plain ▽Sesame			
Quaker	Popcorn cakes: ▽White cheddar Rice cakes: ▽Plain ▽Wheat cakes			
Ralston			Chex snack mix: Traditional	Chex snack mix: *Cool sour cream and onion* Golden cheddar cheese
Rokeach				Dutch pretzels: *No salt added* Regular
Ruffles			Light potato chips: Original Potato chips: Mesquite grille BBQ Original	Light potato chips: Sour cream and onion Potato chips: Cheddar and sour cream Ranch
S & W			Shoestring potatoes	
Sanitas			▽Lightly salted tortilla chips	
Skinny Haven	Skinny munchies: ▽Crispy chocolate treats ▽Smoky BBQ			Skinny munchies: Nacho cheese

▽ Low sodium, 140 mg. or less per serving.

BRAND	ACCEPTABLE			NOT RECOMMENDED
	Without added fat and/or lowfat, 2 grams fat or less per 1 ounce serving (may be partially hydrogenated) may be high in sodium	With added unsaturated oil most are high in fat and sodium (LIMIT USE)	With added acceptable partially hydrogenated oil or shortening most are high in fat and sodium (LIMIT USE)	With added saturated fat
Skinny Haven (Cont'd)	Skinny munchies (Cont'd): ▽Toasted onion			
Snack Time	Pretzels: ▲Butter petite ▲Petite ▲Rods ▲Stix ▲Twist		Indian corn chips Pepitos: Jalapeño flavor Taco ▽Traditional	Baked Cornies cheese puffs Fried Cornies corn puffs Pepitos: Crispy triangle nacho cheese Jalapeño and cheese Nacho cheese
Snyder's of Hanover	Hard pretzels: ▲Sourdough ▽Unsalted sourdough			
Stella D'oro			Breadsticks: ▽Dietetic Plain Sesame Wheat Garlic sticks Onion sticks Sesame sticks	
Wege	▲Dutch pretzels			Pretzels: *Thins*
Weight Watchers			Great snackers: Barbecue	Great snackers: Cheddar cheese

▲ High sodium, 400 mg. or greater per serving.
▽ Low sodium, 140 mg. or less per serving.

Cookies and Fruit Bars

■ **Fat free or contains acceptable oil, 30% or less calories from fat (LIMIT USE)**
Selections from this category are preferred because they contain the least amount of fat. Most of these foods are high in simple sugars and should be consumed only in limited amounts.

◻ **With acceptable partially hydrogenated oil or shortening, 30% or less calories from fat (LIMIT USE)**
Selections from this category are also lower in fat but contain hydrogenated oils. Additionally, they are high in simple sugars and should only be consumed in limited amounts.

◻ **With acceptable oil, hydrogenated oil or shortening, more than 30% calories from fat or unknown amount of fat (LIMIT USE)**
Selections from this category are least desirable. These products contain a higher fat content or the fat content is not known due to missing nutrition labeling. As with all other products in this section, they are high in simple sugars and should only be consumed in limited amounts.

NOT RECOMMENDED

■ **With added saturated fat**
Cookies and fruit bars with added saturated fat are not recommended.

NOTE

■ The approximate sodium content of a serving from this section ranges between 10-120 mg. Sodium symbols are used to indicate high (▲) or low (▽) sodium **only** when sodium content is provided on the product label. Those products that are not identified with either symbol may be either high or low sodium or contain between 141-399 mg. sodium per serving.

BRAND	ACCEPTABLE			NOT RECOMMENDED
	Fat free or contains acceptable oil, 30% or less calories from fat (LIMIT USE)	With acceptable partially hydrogenated oil or shortening, 30% or less calories from fat (LIMIT USE)	With acceptable oil, hydrogenated oil or shortening, more than 30% calories from fat or unknown amount of fat (LIMIT USE)	With added saturated fat
Archway		•Apple 'n Raisin ▽•Apple filled oatmeal ▽•Date filled oatmeal ▽Gingersnaps ▽•Oatmeal Raisin bran •Old fashioned molasses cookies ▽•Ruth's golden oatmeal cookie	•*Almond shortbread* Carrot cake •*Dutch cocoa* Frosty lemon cookie Molasses cookies •*New Orleans cake* •Oatmeal cookies •Oatmeal raisin Old fashioned spice cookies •Peanut butter cookie •Pecan ice box ▽•*Raisin filled oatmeal* •Sugar cookies ▽Windmill cookies	Blueberry filled cookies Cherry filled cookies Chocolate chip: Pack -n- Snack *Chocolate chip and toffee* Chocolate chip cookies Chocolate chip ice box Iced ginger Oatmeal pecan Peanut butter 'n' chips Pineapple filled cookies Raspberry filled cookies Rocky Road Strawberry filled cookies

Awrey's Best	Cholesterol free lowfat:
	  ▲Country bran muffins
		Cholesterol free lowfat:
		  ▽Chocolate loaf cake
		  ▽Golden loaf cake
		Country blueberry muffins
			•*Date nut bars*
			•*Date oatmeal pastries*
			Raisin oatbran cookies
				Cholesterol free lowfat:
				  Apple cinnamon coffee cake
				  Cheese coffee cake
				  Pineapple cheese coffee cake
				  Raspberry coffee cake
				Dutch chocolate chip cookies
				Fudge nut brownie cookies

▲ High sodium, 400 mg. or greater per serving.
▽ Low sodium, 140 mg. or less per serving.
• Contains egg yolks.

Brand	Acceptable			Not Recommended
	Fat free or contains acceptable oil, 30% or less calories from fat (LIMIT USE)	With acceptable partially hydrogenated oil or shortening, 30% or less calories from fat (LIMIT USE)	With acceptable oil, hydrogenated oil or shortening, more than 30% calories from fat or unknown amount of fat (LIMIT USE)	With added saturated fat

Bahlsen			*Bambini cookies*	*Apple crumblies*
				 Choco leibniz:
				   Bittersweet chocolate
				   Milk chocolate
				 Choco-Star
				 Delice
				 Leibniz butter cookies
				 Mokka-Ariba
				 Probiers
				 Strawberry crumblies
				 Waffletten:
				   Milk chocolate
				   Plain

Barbara's	Fruit and nut cookies
	 Oatmeal raisin cookies
				Animal cookies:
				   Carob
				   Chocolate
				   Cinnamon
				   Vanilla
				 Chocolate chip cookies
				 French vanilla cookies
				 Fudge cremes
				 Lemon cremes
				 Vanilla cremes

BRAND	ACCEPTABLE			NOT RECOMMENDED
	Fat free or contains acceptable oil, 30% or less calories from fat (LIMIT USE)	With acceptable partially hydrogenated oil or shortening, 30% or less calories from fat (LIMIT USE)	With acceptable oil, hydrogenated oil or shortening, more than 30% calories from fat or unknown amount of fat (LIMIT USE)	With added saturated fat
Betty Crocker		Fruit roll-ups: ▽*Grape* ▽Raspberry ▽Strawberry Fruit wrinkles: ▽Cherry ▽Grape ▽Orange ▽Strawberry ▽Watermelon Garfield chewy fruit snacks: ▽1-2 punch ▽Fruit party ▽Very strawberry ▽Wild blueberry ▽Nintendo real fruit snacks ▽Super Mario Brothers real fruit snacks		
Big Value			▽Apple bars Artificially flavored: Chocolate Lemon Oatmeal Fig bars	*Butter cookies* Chocolate chip cookies *Chocolate chip cookies (100 per bag)* Lemon cookies Sugar cookies

▽ Low sodium, 140 mg. or less per serving.

BRAND	ACCEPTABLE			NOT RECOMMENDED
	Fat free or contains acceptable oil, 30% or less calories from fat (LIMIT USE)	With acceptable partially hydrogenated oil or shortening, 30% or less calories from fat (LIMIT USE)	With acceptable oil, hydrogenated oil or shortening, more than 30% calories from fat or unknown amount of fat (LIMIT USE)	With added saturated fat
Big Value (Cont'd)			▽Oatmeal cookies Sandwich cremes: 　Chocolate 　Duplex 　Lemon 　Vanilla Vanilla wafers	
Carnation				Breakfast bars: 　Chocolate chip 　Peanut butter crunch 　Peanut butter with 　　chocolate chip
Carr's				Sesame honey delights
Country Oven		▽Chocolate animal fun cookies	Animal crackers ▽Assorted sugar wafers Cookies 'n Creme: 　*Oatmeal* 　*Vanilla* Gingersnaps ▽*Olde Southern pecan* ▽Prehistoric dinosaur honey graham cookies ▽Sugar wafers ▽Vanilla wafers ▽Waffle cremes	6 in one cookie assortment *Assorted creme wafers* Chip Mates: 　Chocolate chip cookies 　Peanut butter chocolate 　　chip *Chips-a-Plenty* *Coconut chocolate chip cookies* Coconut macaroon cookies Cookies 'n Creme: 　*Chippies*

▽ Low sodium, 140 mg. or less per serving.

BRAND	ACCEPTABLE			NOT RECOMMENDED
	Fat free or contains acceptable oil, 30% or less calories from fat (LIMIT USE)	With acceptable partially hydrogenated oil or shortening, 30% or less calories from fat (LIMIT USE)	With acceptable oil, hydrogenated oil or shortening, more than 30% calories from fat or unknown amount of fat (LIMIT USE)	With added saturated fat
Country Oven (Cont'd)				Cookies 'n Creme (Cont'd): *Combo* *Fudge* Creme wafer sticks Fancy whirls *Fig bars* Fudge chocolate chip Fudge graham cookies *Graham squares* Mint tiara sandwich cremes *Oatmeal chocolate chip cookies* Peanut butter animal crackers Peanut butter chocolate chip *Peanut butter cookie patties* *Peanut butter creme wafer sticks* Sandwich cremes: Deluxe tiara Mint tiara Striped Royales Windmill cookies
De Beukelaer Corporation				*Pirouluxe*

BRAND	**ACCEPTABLE**			**NOT RECOMMENDED**
	Fat free or contains acceptable oil, 30% or less calories from fat (LIMIT USE)	With acceptable partially hydrogenated oil or shortening, 30% or less calories from fat (LIMIT USE)	With acceptable oil, hydrogenated oil or shortening, more than 30% calories from fat or unknown amount of fat (LIMIT USE)	With added saturated fat

Del Monte				Fruit snacks:
				   Original yogurt raisins
				   Sierra trail mix
				   Strawberry yogurt, raisins

Duncan Hines				Chocolate chip cookies

El Molino			Animal cookies:
			   Carob honey
			   Ginger honey
			   Graham honey
			   Honey	

Entenmann's	Fat free cholesterol free:
	  ▽Apple cinnamon twist
	  ▽Banana crunch cake
	  ▽Cheese filled crumb
	    coffee cake
	  ▽Chocolate loaf cake
	  ▽Cinnamon apple
	    coffee cake
	  ▽Fruit and honey
	    cookies
	  ▽Golden loaf cake
	  ▽Lemon twist
	  ▽Oatmeal raisin
	    cookies
			•Oat bran raisin
			Oatmeal raisin and nut
				Butter cookies
				Chocolate chip
				Crispy chocolate chip
				English toffee cookies
				Gourmet butter cookies

▽ Low sodium, 140 mg. or less per serving.
• Contains egg yolks.

BRAND	ACCEPTABLE			NOT RECOMMENDED
	Fat free or contains acceptable oil, 30% or less calories from fat (LIMIT USE)	With acceptable partially hydrogenated oil or shortening, 30% or less calories from fat (LIMIT USE)	With acceptable oil, hydrogenated oil or shortening, more than 30% calories from fat or unknown amount of fat (LIMIT USE)	With added saturated fat
Entenmann's (Cont'd)	▽Fat free oatmeal raisin cookies			

Estee		▽Fudge cookies
		▽Lemon thins
		▽Oatmeal raisin cookies
		▽Vanilla thins
			Cremes filled wafer sugar free:
			  ▽Assorted
			  ▽Chocolate
			▽Original sandwich cookies
			Sandwich cookies:
			  ▽Chocolate
			  ▽Original
			  ▽Peanut butter
				Chocolate chip
				Coconut cookies
				Cremes filled wafer sugar free:
				  Vanilla

Farley's	Fruit snacks:
	  ▽Cherry
	  Dinosaurs
	  ▽Grape
	  ▽Strawberry
	  Teenage Mutant Ninja Turtles			

Featherweight			Sweet Pretenders:
			  ▽Vanilla
				Sweet Pretenders:
				  Chocolate flavored chip cookies

▽ Low sodium, 140 mg. or less per serving.

BRAND	ACCEPTABLE			NOT RECOMMENDED
	Fat free or contains acceptable oil, 30% or less calories from fat (LIMIT USE)	With acceptable partially hydrogenated oil or shortening, 30% or less calories from fat (LIMIT USE)	With acceptable oil, hydrogenated oil or shortening, more than 30% calories from fat or unknown amount of fat (LIMIT USE)	With added saturated fat
Fruit Corners		Shark bites: ▽Assorted fruit ▽Fruit punch The Berry Bears chewy fruit snacks: ▽Assorted ▽Fruit punch ▽Thunder jets		
Fruit Sweet			▽Oatmeal cookies ▽Peanut butter cookies	Coconut macaroons
Gateway Bakery			Cookies 'n Creme sandwich cookies: Oatmeal Vanilla	Cookies 'n Creme sandwich cookies: Chippies Combo Fudge
Health Valley	Fancy fruit chunks: ▽Raisin oat bran ▽Tropical fruit		100% Natural fruit bars: ▽★Apple bakes ▽Date bakes	

▽ Low sodium, 140 mg. or less per serving.
★ High fiber, 3 g. or greater per serving.

BRAND	ACCEPTABLE			NOT RECOMMENDED
	Fat free or contains acceptable oil, 30% or less calories from fat (LIMIT USE)	With acceptable partially hydrogenated oil or shortening, 30% or less calories from fat (LIMIT USE)	With acceptable oil, hydrogenated oil or shortening, more than 30% calories from fat or unknown amount of fat (LIMIT USE)	With added saturated fat

Health Valley (Cont'd)	▽Fancy peanut chunks peanut butter
	Fat free:
	  Apple spice cookies
	  Date delight cookies
	Fruit jumbos:
	  ▽Oat bran
	Honey jumbos:
	  ▽★*Fancy oat bran*
	  ▽Peanut butter crisp
	Jumbo fruit bars:
	  Raisin and cinnamon
	▽★Oat bran graham crackers
	Oatbran jumbo fruit bars:
	  ▽★Date and almond
	  ▽★Fruit and nut
	  Raisin and cinnamon
	  ▽★Rice bran with almonds and dates
			100% Natural fruit bars (Cont'd):
			  ▽*Raisin bakes*
			Fancy fruit chunks:
			  ▽Apricot almond
			  ▽Date pecan
			▽Fruit and nut oat bran cookies
			Fruit jumbos:
			  ▽Almond date
			  ▽Raisin nut
			  ▽Tropical fruit
			Honey jumbos:
			  ▽Cinnamon crisp
			  ▽*Oat bran crisp*
			▽Oat bran animal cookies	

Hostess		Cupcakes Lights Twinkies Lights		
Jack LaLanne				Fruit and nut granola bars: Apple nut

▽ Low sodium, 140 mg. or less per serving.
★ High fiber, 3 g. or greater per serving.

BRAND	ACCEPTABLE			NOT RECOMMENDED
	Fat free or contains acceptable oil, 30% or less calories from fat (LIMIT USE)	With acceptable partially hydrogenated oil or shortening, 30% or less calories from fat (LIMIT USE)	With acceptable oil, hydrogenated oil or shortening, more than 30% calories from fat or unknown amount of fat (LIMIT USE)	With added saturated fat
Jack LaLanne (Cont'd)				Fruit and nut granola bars (Cont'd): Banana nut Date nut
Keebler		▽Iced animal cookies	Magic middles: Crisp oatmeal ▽•Shortbread ▽•Walnut fudge Mini middles: Oatmeal Shortbread Original cookie classics: ▽French vanilla creme ▽Oatmeal cremes ▽Pitter Patter ▽•Pecan sandies ▽Playland cookies Soft batch: Oatmeal raisin ▽Peanut butter nut	Baby bear cookies Chips Deluxe Coconut chocolate drop Deluxe grahams Double dominoes E.L. Fudge: Butter flavored cookie with fudge creme filling Fudge cookies with fudge creme filling Fudge cookies with peanut butter creme filling Fudge cookies with vanilla creme filling Fudge covered buttery cookie Elfkins: Butter cookies with fudge filling Fudge cookies with fudge filling

▽ Low sodium, 140 mg. or less per serving.
• Contains egg yolks.

BRAND	ACCEPTABLE			NOT RECOMMENDED
	Fat free or contains acceptable oil, 30% or less calories from fat (LIMIT USE)	With acceptable partially hydrogenated oil or shortening, 30% or less calories from fat (LIMIT USE)	With acceptable oil, hydrogenated oil or shortening, more than 30% calories from fat or unknown amount of fat (LIMIT USE)	With added saturated fat
Keebler (Cont'd)				Fudge dominoes: *Chocolate cookies with white fudge* *Graham cookie with chocolate fudge* Fudge sticks Fudge stripes Golden vanilla wafers Grasshopper Magic middles: Chocolate chip Mini middles: Chocolate chip Original cookie classics: Chocolate fudge *Grasshopper* Rainbow chips deluxe Soft batch: Chocolate chip *Peanut butter chocolate chip* Walnut chocolate chip
Kellogg's				Rice Krispies bars: Chocolate chip *Peanut butter*

BRAND	ACCEPTABLE			NOT RECOMMENDED
	Fat free or contains acceptable oil, 30% or less calories from fat (LIMIT USE)	With acceptable partially hydrogenated oil or shortening, 30% or less calories from fat (LIMIT USE)	With acceptable oil, hydrogenated oil or shortening, more than 30% calories from fat or unknown amount of fat (LIMIT USE)	With added saturated fat
Kremini				Cookies with hazelnut cream filling
Kroger		Box o Bears: ▽Chocolate ▽Cinnamon ▽Honey ▽Fruit snack dinosaurs Fruit snacks: ▽Cherry ▽Sharks ▽Strawberry ▽Variety pack	▽Old Southern pecan cookies	Caramel and chocolate chips Chewy granola bars: *Chocolate chip* *Peanut butter* Chip mates: Chocolate chip cookies Peanut butter and chocolate chip cookies Chips-a-plenty: Caramel and chocolate chip Chocolate fudge covered cookies
Kudos				Chocolate and granola snacks: *Butter almond* Chocolate chip Cookies and creme Crunchy nut Nutty fudge Peanut butter Raisin

▽ Low sodium, 140 mg. or less per serving.

BRAND	ACCEPTABLE			NOT RECOMMENDED
	Fat free or contains acceptable oil, 30% or less calories from fat (LIMIT USE)	With acceptable partially hydrogenated oil or shortening, 30% or less calories from fat (LIMIT USE)	With acceptable oil, hydrogenated oil or shortening, more than 30% calories from fat or unknown amount of fat (LIMIT USE)	With added saturated fat
La Choy		Fortune cookies		
Little Debbie			▽Fudge crispy Lemon stix •Marshmallow supremes ▽Nutty bar •Peanut butter bars Strawberry wafers	Apple delights Oatmeal creme pies Star crunch
Matilde's				Egg biscuits Puff pastries
Mi-Del	Honey grahams			

Motor City Muffins			Cookies:
			  Partner oat bran
				Cookies:
				  Cowgirl oatmeal chocolate chip

Nabisco		Newtons:
		  •Apple
		  Fig
		  •Raspberry
		  •Strawberry
		Teddy grahams:
		  Cinnamon
		  Honey
		  Vanilla
			Almost Home:
			  •Oatmeal raisin
			  •Sugar
			Cameo
			Cookies and fudge:
			  Striped wafers
			•Lorna Doone
			•Nutter Butter
			•Pecan shortbread
			Suddenly S'mores
				'Nilla wafers
				Almost Home:
				  Chocolate fudge chip
				  Peanut butter fudge
				  Real chocolate chip
				  Walnut chocolate chip
				Barnum's Animal crackers
				Chewy Chips Ahoy
				Chips Ahoy
				Chips Ahoy selections:
				  Chunky

▽ Low sodium, 140 mg. or less per serving.
• Contains egg yolks.

BRAND	ACCEPTABLE			NOT RECOMMENDED
	Fat free or contains acceptable oil, 30% or less calories from fat (LIMIT USE)	With acceptable partially hydrogenated oil or shortening, 30% or less calories from fat (LIMIT USE)	With acceptable oil, hydrogenated oil or shortening, more than 30% calories from fat or unknown amount of fat (LIMIT USE)	With added saturated fat
Nabisco (Cont'd)				Chips Ahoy selections (Cont'd): Chunky chocolate chip Oatmeal chocolate chunk Cookies and fudge: Party grahams *Striped chocolate chip* *Striped peanut butter nut* Striped shortbread Devil's food cakes *Famous chocolate wafers* Fudge covered oreo Ginger snaps Marshmallow twirls Oreo: Big Stuff Double Stuff Regular Sprinkled Chips Ahoy Striped Chips Ahoy Teddy grahams: Chocolate
Natural Nectar	Fi-Bar: ▽★Mandarin Orange ▽★Raspberry	Fi-Bar: ▽★Apple	Fi-Bar: ▽★Lemon	Fi-Bar, Chewy and nutty: Cocoa almond crunch Cocoa peanut crunch

▽ Low sodium, 140 mg. or less per serving.
★ High fiber, 3 g. or greater per serving.

BRAND	ACCEPTABLE			NOT RECOMMENDED
	Fat free or contains acceptable oil, 30% or less calories from fat (LIMIT USE)	With acceptable partially hydrogenated oil or shortening, 30% or less calories from fat (LIMIT USE)	With acceptable oil, hydrogenated oil or shortening, more than 30% calories from fat or unknown amount of fat (LIMIT USE)	With added saturated fat
Natural Nectar (Cont'd)		Fi-Bar (Cont'd): ▽★Cranberry & wild berries ▽★Strawberry		Fi-Bar, Chewy and nutty (Cont'd): Vanilla almond crunch Vanilla peanut crunch
Nature Valley			Granola bars: ▽Oats 'n Honey	
Nature's Choice	Fresh and chewy granola bars: ▽Carob chip ▽Cinnamon and raisin ▽Oats and honey Oat bran bars: ▽Cinnamon apple ▽Mixed fruit ▽Triple bran with apricots Real fruit bars: ▽Apricot ▽Cherry ▽Grape ▽Raspberry		Fresh and chewy granola bars: ▽Peanut butter	
Nature's Warehouse	Pastry poppers: ▽Apple ▽Blueberry		Wheat free almond butter cookie	

▽ Low sodium, 140 mg. or less per serving.
★ High fiber, 3 g. or greater per serving.

BRAND	ACCEPTABLE			NOT RECOMMENDED
	Fat free or contains acceptable oil, 30% or less calories from fat (LIMIT USE)	With acceptable partially hydrogenated oil or shortening, 30% or less calories from fat (LIMIT USE)	With acceptable oil, hydrogenated oil or shortening, more than 30% calories from fat or unknown amount of fat (LIMIT USE)	With added saturated fat
Nature's Warehouse (Cont'd)	Pastry poppers (Cont'd): ▽Peach apricot ▽Raspberry			
Nestle				Raisinets
Pastry Shoppe			•40 sugar cookies ▽Oat bran raisin •Peanut butter cookies •Pecan crisp •Sugar cookies	40 chocolate chip cookies Butter brickle Chocolate candy Chocolate chip Gourmet chocolate chip pecan cookies Gourmet honey nut raisin Heath bar Oatmeal cookies Peanut butter Peanut candy cookie
Peek Freans				Arrowroot biscuits *Assorted biscuits* *Dark chocolate biscuits* Fruit creme biscuits Ginger crisp biscuits Milk chocolate biscuits Nice biscuits Petit Beurre biscuits

▽ Low sodium, 140 mg. or less per serving.
• Contains egg yolks.

BRAND	ACCEPTABLE			NOT RECOMMENDED
	Fat free or contains acceptable oil, 30% or less calories from fat (LIMIT USE)	With acceptable partially hydrogenated oil or shortening, 30% or less calories from fat (LIMIT USE)	With acceptable oil, hydrogenated oil or shortening, more than 30% calories from fat or unknown amount of fat (LIMIT USE)	With added saturated fat
Peek Freans (Cont'd)				Rich tea biscuits Shortcake biscuits Sweetmeal biscuits
Pepperidge Farm			American collection: •Santa Fe •Ginger man cookies •Hazelnut cookies •Irish oatmeal cookies Molasses crisps Original pirouettes	American collection: Beacon hill Chesapeake Dakota Nantucket Sausalito Apricot raspberry fruit cookie Bordeaux cookies Brownie chocolate nut Brussels cookies Brussels mint cookies Capri brownie cream cookies Champagne cookie collection Chessman butter cookies Chocolate chip Chocolate chunk pecan Chocolate laced pirouettes Date pecan cookies Lido cookies Linzer cookies Milano cookies

• Contains egg yolks.

BRAND	ACCEPTABLE			NOT RECOMMENDED
	Fat free or contains acceptable oil, 30% or less calories from fat (LIMIT USE)	With acceptable partially hydrogenated oil or shortening, 30% or less calories from fat (LIMIT USE)	With acceptable oil, hydrogenated oil or shortening, more than 30% calories from fat or unknown amount of fat (LIMIT USE)	With added saturated fat
Pepperidge Farm (Cont'd)				Nassau cookies Orange Mikino cookies Orleans sandwich cookies Seville cookie collection Shortbread cookies Southport cookie collection Sugar cookies Tahiti cookies
Quaker				Chewy granola bars: Apple Chocolate chip Chunky nut and raisin Peanut butter and chocolate chip Strawberry Granola dipps: Caramel nut Chocolate chip Chocolate fudge Peanut butter chocolate chip
R.W. Frookie		Animal frackers	▽7-grain oatmeal ▽Apple cinnamon oat bran	Mandarin orange chocolate chip *Mint chocolate chip*

▽ Low sodium, 140 mg. or less per serving.

BRAND	ACCEPTABLE			NOT RECOMMENDED
	Fat free or contains acceptable oil, 30% or less calories from fat (LIMIT USE)	With acceptable partially hydrogenated oil or shortening, 30% or less calories from fat (LIMIT USE)	With acceptable oil, hydrogenated oil or shortening, more than 30% calories from fat or unknown amount of fat (LIMIT USE)	With added saturated fat
R.W. Frookie (Cont'd)			▽Ginger spice ▽Oat bran muffin cookie ▽Oatmeal raisin	
Salerno			•Dinosaur grahams Mini dinosaur grahams: 　•Cinnamon 　•Original	Mini dinosaur grahams: 　Chocolate
Stella D'oro	•Almond toast •Anisette sponge •Anisette toast		•*Angel wings* •*Angelica goodies* •Anginetti •Breakfast treats •Chinese dessert cookies •Chocolate castelets •Deep night fudge cookies ▽•Dietetic apple pastry •*Dietetic egg biscuit* •Golden bars •Margherite •Margherite combination •Roman egg biscuits •Sesame cookies	*Angel bars* *Dutch apple bars* Lady Stella assortment Swiss fudge cookies

▽ Low sodium, 140 mg. or less per serving.
• Contains egg yolks.

BRAND	ACCEPTABLE			NOT RECOMMENDED
	Fat free or contains acceptable oil, 30% or less calories from fat (LIMIT USE)	With acceptable partially hydrogenated oil or shortening, 30% or less calories from fat (LIMIT USE)	With acceptable oil, hydrogenated oil or shortening, more than 30% calories from fat or unknown amount of fat (LIMIT USE)	With added saturated fat
Sunkist		Fruit rox: ▽Galactic gems Fun fruits: ▽Animals ▽Berry punch ▽Cherry ▽Dinosaurs ▽Letters ▽Numbers ▽Space shapes ▽Spooky fruits ▽Strawberry ▽Strawberry banana Two-t-Fruits: ▽Cherry 'n Grape ▽Strawberry 'n Cherry ▽Strawberry 'n Grape		Fruit rox: Meteorites
Sunshine		▽•Golden fruit raisin biscuits	Country style oatmeal cookies Fudge family bears: Chocolate Peanut butter filled Vanilla	Bavarian fingers Butter flavored cookies Chip-a-roos Chocolate cookiesaurus Fudge family bears: Peanut butter

▽ Low sodium, 140 mg. or less per serving.
• Contains egg yolks.

BRAND	ACCEPTABLE			NOT RECOMMENDED
	Fat free or contains acceptable oil, 30% or less calories from fat (LIMIT USE)	With acceptable partially hydrogenated oil or shortening, 30% or less calories from fat (LIMIT USE)	With acceptable oil, hydrogenated oil or shortening, more than 30% calories from fat or unknown amount of fat (LIMIT USE)	With added saturated fat
Sunshine (Cont'd)			Grahamy bears O.T. Bears ▽ *Vienna fingers*	Hydrox Vanilla wafers

Thompson Foods			Ideal bars:
			  ▽★*Date-n-Orange*
			  ▽★*Green apple*
			  ▽★*Peaches and spice*
				Ideal bars:
				  Cherry coconut almond
				  Raspberry
				  Tropical fruit

Twix				*Caramel cookie bars* Peanut butter cookie bars
UMEYA		Fortune cookies		
Voortman			•Almond krunch •Almonettes Double fudge •Oatmeal apple •Shortbread swirl •Sugar cookies	Almond speculaas Brownie nut Chocolate chips Dutch creme cookies Fudge swirls Gingerboys Graham bears Oatmeal chip Peanut delight Windmill cookies

▽ Low sodium, 140 mg. or less per serving.
★ High fiber, 3 g. or greater per serving.
• Contains egg yolks.

BRAND	ACCEPTABLE			NOT RECOMMENDED
	Fat free or contains acceptable oil, 30% or less calories from fat (LIMIT USE)	With acceptable partially hydrogenated oil or shortening, 30% or less calories from fat (LIMIT USE)	With acceptable oil, hydrogenated oil or shortening, more than 30% calories from fat or unknown amount of fat (LIMIT USE)	With added saturated fat
Weight Watchers	Fruit snacks: ▽Apple ▽Cinnamon ▽Peach			
Zion			Whole wheat fig bars	Oatmeal and date bars
REFRIGERATED & FROZEN COOKIE DOUGH:				
Nestle Toll House				Frozen brownie batter: *Double chocolate chip* Frozen cookie dough: Chocolate chip Chocolate chip with nuts *Double chocolate chip* Oatmeal raisin
Pillsbury's Best			•Peanut butter cookies ▽•Sugar cookies	Chocolate chip cookies Chocolate chocolate chip cookies Oatmeal raisin cookies

▽ Low sodium, 140 mg. or less per serving.
• Contains egg yolks.

Crackers

■ **Without added fat**

These crackers are preferred choices because they do not contain added fats and are therefore lower in calories.

▨ **With added unsaturated oil (LIMIT USE),** and

▨ **With added acceptable partially hydrogenated oil or shortening (LIMIT USE)**

Crackers listed in this and the preceding category contain added acceptable fats. Most selections are high in fat and therefore high in calories. Crackers that are known to contain greater than 2 grams fat per serving are identified with a (†) symbol. Limited use is recommended.

NOT RECOMMENDED

■ **With added saturated fat**

Crackers with added saturated fat are not recommended.

NOTE

■ The sodium content of crackers is variable depending on the amount of added salt. Low salt snack crackers contain approximately 40-95 mg. sodium per ½ ounce serving, whereas salted crackers may contain as much as 210 mg. per ½ ounce serving. Sodium symbols are used to indicate high (▲) or low (▽) sodium **only** when sodium content is provided on the product label. Those products that are not identified with either symbol may be either high or low sodium or contain between 141-399 mg. sodium per serving.

BRAND	ACCEPTABLE			NOT RECOMMENDED
	Without added fat	With added unsaturated oil (LIMIT USE)	With added acceptable partially hydrogenated oil or shortening (LIMIT USE)	With added saturated fat
Ak-Mak				100% Stone-ground crackers
Bi-Rite				*Saltines*
Carr's				Assorted biscuits for cheese Croissant crackers Sesame honey delights Table water crackers Table water crackers with sesame seeds Whole wheat crackers
Cost Cutter			Saltines ▽Snack crackers	Graham crackers
Estee			▽Unsalted snack crackers ▽Wheat wafers	
Famous Foods of Virginia	*Sesame crisp wafers*		†*Roman meal wafers* ▲*Stoned wheat wafers*	
First for Value			▽Sesame crisp wafers	
Hain Naturals		Stoneground wheat: ▽†Onion crackers, no salt added ▽Rye crackers ▽†Sesame crackers ▽†Vegetable crackers		Stoneground wheat: Cheese crackers
Health Valley		▽†*Fancy honey grahams*		

▲ High sodium, 400 mg. or greater per serving.
▽ Low sodium, 140 mg. or less per serving.
† High fat, contains greater than 2 g. fat per serving. Limit use.

BRAND	ACCEPTABLE			NOT RECOMMENDED
	Without added fat	With added unsaturated oil (LIMIT USE)	With added acceptable partially hydrogenated oil or shortening (LIMIT USE)	With added saturated fat
Health Valley (Cont'd)		▽★†Herb stoned wheat crackers †Sesame stoned wheat crackers ▽★†Stoned wheat crackers ▽★†Oat bran graham crackers		
Hol-Ry Old Country				Zwieback: Cinnamon Plain
Jacobsen's			▽Cinnamon snack toast	
Kavli	Norwegian crispbread: ▽Thick style ▽Thin style			
Keebler	Whole wheat Jrs.		▽†Chocolate graham thin bits ▽Cinnamon crisp grahams ▽†Cinnamon graham thin bits Club crackers: ▽†Low salt †Regular ▽Honey grahams	Club and cheddar cracker sandwiches Cracker sandwiches: Cheese and peanut butter Wheat and American cheese Harvest wheats Honey grahams thin bits Munch 'ems: Cheddar

▽ Low sodium, 140 mg. or less per serving.
★ High fiber, 3 g. or greater per serving.
† High fat, contains greater than 2 g. fat per serving. Limit use.

BRAND	ACCEPTABLE			NOT RECOMMENDED
	Without added fat	With added unsaturated oil (LIMIT USE)	With added acceptable partially hydrogenated oil or shortening (LIMIT USE)	With added saturated fat

Keebler (Cont'd)			Munch 'ems:
			  †Original
			  †Sour cream and onion
			Stone creek:
			  ▽*Hearty rye*
			▽†Sun Toasted wheats
			Toasteds:
			  ▽†Bacon
			  ▽†Onion
			  ▽†Rye
			  ▽†Sesame
			  ▽†Wheat
			Townhouse:
			  ▽†Bite Size Jrs.
			  ▽†Low salt Classic crackers
			  ▽†Regular Classic crackers
			Wheatables:
			  ▽†Low salt
			  ▽†Whole wheat snacks
			Zesta:
			  ▽Low salt
			  Original
			  Wheat
			  Wheat saltine crackers
				Stone creek:
				  Cracked wheat
				Toasteds:
				  Buttercrisp
				Townhouse:
				  Cheddar cheese Jrs.
				  Cheddar cheese snacks
				  Whole wheat Jrs.
				TUCs
				Wheatables:
				  Ranch flavor
				  White cheddar flavor
				Zesta:
				  Unsalted tops

Kraft			Handi snacks:
			  Peanut butter 'n Cheez
				Handi snacks:
				  Bacon Cheez 'n Crackers
				  Cheez 'n Crackers

▽ Low sodium, 140 mg. or less per serving.
† High fat, contains greater than 2 g. fat per serving. Limit use.

BRAND	ACCEPTABLE			NOT RECOMMENDED
	Without added fat	With added unsaturated oil (LIMIT USE)	With added acceptable partially hydrogenated oil or shortening (LIMIT USE)	With added saturated fat
Kroger			▽†Country Club Crackers (saltines) ▽Honey graham ▽Low salt saltines ▽†Oat squares ▽Original graham crackers Oyster crackers: 　Regular 　▽Unsalted tops Saltines ▽Socialites ▽Unsalted top crackers ▽Wheat saltines Wheat squares: 　▽†Low salt 　▽Nutty 　▽†Oat 　▽†Original Zips: 　▽†Low salt 　▽†Regular Zips Bitz: 　▽†Low salt	Cheese bits: 　Low salt 　Regular Cheese on cheese 　sandwiches Cheese thins: 　Cheddar 　Cheddar and bacon 　*Swiss* Cinnamon and raisin 　grahams Cinnamon graham crackers Light and crispy: 　*French onion* 　*Real bacon* 　*Sesame* Oyster crackers: 　Cheese Oyster crisps *Stone ground wheat crackers* *Stone ground wheat sesame* 　*crackers* Toasty peanut butter 　sandwiches Wheat rounds Zips Bitz: 　Regular

▽ Low sodium, 140 mg. or less per serving.
† High fat, contains greater than 2 g. fat per serving. Limit use.

BRAND	ACCEPTABLE			NOT RECOMMENDED
	Without added fat	With added unsaturated oil (LIMIT USE)	With added acceptable partially hydrogenated oil or shortening (LIMIT USE)	With added saturated fat

Manischewitz	Matzos:
	▽•Dietetic Matzo Thins
	•Egg and Onion
	▽Matzo-cracker
	  miniatures
	Thin Salted
	▽Thin Tea
	▽Unsalted
	▽★Whole wheat
				Crackers:
				  Garlic Tams
				  Onion Tams
				  Tam Tam

Master Old Country	★Natural grain hardtack		▽Zwieback plain toast	
Mi-Del		100% whole wheat honey grahams		

Nabisco	▽Fat Free Premium crackers		American Classics:
			  Cracked wheat
			  Dairy butter
			  Golden sesame
			  Toasted poppy
			▽†Chicken in a Biskit
			▽†Escort
			Harvest Crisps:
			  ▽Oat crackers
			Honey Maid:
			  ▽Cinnamon grahams
			▽†Oat thins
				Bacon flavored crackers
				Better Cheddars:
				  Bacon
				  Low salt
				  Regular
				Cheese Tid-Bits
				Dandy soup and oyster
				  crackers
				Doo dads snack mix
				Honey Maid:
				  Honey grahams
				Nabisco grahams

▽ Low sodium, 140 mg. or less per serving.
• Contains egg yolks.
★ High fiber, 3 g. or greater per serving.
† High fat, contains greater than 2 g. fat per serving. Limit use.

BRAND	ACCEPTABLE			NOT RECOMMENDED
	Without added fat	With added unsaturated oil (LIMIT USE)	With added acceptable partially hydrogenated oil or shortening (LIMIT USE)	With added saturated fat

Nabisco (Cont'd)			†Premium Bits
			Premium Plus:
			  ▽Whole wheat
			Premium saltines:
			  ▽Low salt
			  Original
			  ▽Unsalted tops
			Ritz bits:
			  ▽†Low salt
			  ▽†Regular
			  ▽†Sandwiches with
			    peanut butter
			▽†Sociables
			Triscuit Bits:
			  ▽Mini-triscuit wafers
			Triscuits:
			  ▽Low salt
			  ▽Original
			  ▽Wheat 'n Bran
			†Waverly
			Wheat Thins:
			  ▽†Low salt
			  †Nutty
			  ▽†Original
			▽†Wheatsworth
				Nips cheese snack crackers:
				  Cheddar cheese
				Quackers:
				  Cheddar cheese
				  Sour cream and onion
				Ritz bits:
				  Cheese
				  Sandwiches with real
				    cheese
				Ritz crackers:
				  Low salt
				  Regular
				Sesame and cheese twigs
				Swiss cheese snack crackers
				Vegetable thins

Old Brussels				*Cheddar cheese snack wafferettes*

▽ Low sodium, 140 mg. or less per serving.
† High fat, contains greater than 2 g. fat per serving. Limit use.

BRAND	ACCEPTABLE			NOT RECOMMENDED
	Without added fat	With added unsaturated oil (LIMIT USE)	With added acceptable partially hydrogenated oil or shortening (LIMIT USE)	With added saturated fat
Old London	Krisp and natural crackerbread: ▽Whole wheat	Krisp and natural crackerbread: ▽Wheat	Melba snacks: ▽Bacon rounds ▽Garlic rounds ▽Onion rounds Sesame rounds ▽White ▽Whole grain Melba toast: ▽Rye ▽Sesame ▽Unsalted white ▽Unsalted whole grain ▽Wheat ▽White ▽Whole grain	
Pepperidge Farm			†Golden sesame flutters Goldfish tiny crackers: †Pizza flavored ▽†Hearty Wheat ▽†Sesame crackers ▽†Toasted wheat ▽†Toasted wheat flutters	Butter flavored thins *Cracked wheat* *English water biscuits* Goldfish tiny crackers: Cheddar cheese Cheddar cheese, low salt Original Symphony cracker assortment
Ralston	▽★Natural Ry-Krisp		▽★†Oatbran Krisp ▽★Seasoned Ry-Krisp	

▽ Low sodium, 140 mg. or less per serving.
★ High fiber, 3 g. or greater per serving.
† High fat, contains greater than 2 g. fat per serving. Limit use.

BRAND	ACCEPTABLE			NOT RECOMMENDED
	Without added fat	With added unsaturated oil (LIMIT USE)	With added acceptable partially hydrogenated oil or shortening (LIMIT USE)	With added saturated fat
Red Oval Farms			Stoned rye crackers Stoned wheat thins	Sesame and onion crackers
Ryvita	▽Tasty light rye	▽★Snack bread		
Streit's		Moonstrips matzos: Onion flavored	Unsalted matzos	

Sunshine			▽†American Heritage crackers
			▽†Cheese Shuffles
			Cheez-it:
			  ▽†Low salt
			  ▽†Regular
			▽†Hi Ho
			▽†Hi Ho Deluxe
			▽†Hi Ho Deluxe low salt crackers
			▽Honey grahams
			Krispy:
			  Original
			  ▽Unsalted tops
			  Whole wheat
			▽†Oat bran heart-shaped snack crackers
			Wheats:
			  †Heart shaped crackers	

▽ Low sodium, 140 mg. or less per serving.
★ High fiber, 3 g. or greater per serving.
† High fat, contains greater than 2 g. fat per serving. Limit use.

BRAND	ACCEPTABLE			NOT RECOMMENDED
	Without added fat	**With added unsaturated oil (LIMIT USE)**	**With added acceptable partially hydrogenated oil or shortening (LIMIT USE)**	**With added saturated fat**
The House of Aulsebrooks			Traditional water crackers	
Venus			*Rye wafers* ▽Salt free bran wafers ▽★*Salt free corn crackers* ▽Salt free cracked wheat wafers *Toasted sesame squares* Wheat wafers	
Wasa	Crispbread: ▽Golden rye ▽Hearty rye ▽Lite rye ▽★Royal wholegrain ▽*Savory sesame*		Crispbread: ▽Breakfast ▽Fiber Plus ▽Sesame wheat ▽Toasted wheat	
Weight Watchers				Crispbread: Garlic Golden wheat
Win Schuler's			Bar Schips: *Bacon* *Garlic* *Natural rye*	Bar Schips: *Sour cream and onion*

▽ Low sodium, 140 mg. or less per serving.
★ High fiber, 3 g. or greater per serving.

Popcorn
(Ready Made)

■ **Plain, without added fat**
Popcorn selections from this category are preferred because they contain no added fat.

■ **With added acceptable partially hydrogenated oil (LIMIT USE)**
Commercially prepared popcorns that contain partially hydrogenated oil are higher in fat (approximately 60% calories from fat). Limited intake is recommended.

NOT RECOMMENDED

■ **With added saturated fat**
Popcorn with added saturated fat is not recommended.

NOTE

■ The sodium content of popcorn varies depending on added salt. Low salt popcorn contains approximately 110 mg. sodium per 1 ounce serving. Regular salted popcorn may contain as much as 240 mg. sodium per 1 ounce serving. Sodium symbols are used to indicate high (▲) or low (▽) sodium **only** when sodium content is provided on the product label. Those products that are not identified with either symbol may be either high or low sodium or contain between 141-399 mg. sodium per serving.

Brand	Acceptable		Not Recommended
	Plain, without added fat	With added acceptable partially hydrogenated oil (LIMIT USE)	With added saturated fat
Big Value			*Cheese flavored popcorn*
Cape Cod			Popcorn: White cheddar cheese
Eagle			Popcorn: White cheddar
Franklin			Crunch n' Munch
Keebler			Deluxe white cheddar

Kroger		Kroger popcorn:
		  ▽*Buttery gourmet, low salt*
		  ▽*Gourmet, low salt*
			Kroger popcorn:
			  Buttery
			  Caramel corn with peanuts
			  Cheese
			  White cheddar cheese

Michael Seasons			Popcorn: White cheddar cheese
Poppy Cock		Popcorn-walnuts-cashews	Popcorn-almonds-pecans
Smartfood			Kentucky popcorn: Cheddar cheese

Snack Time		Popcorn:
		  Fresh popped flavor
		  Whole white kernels
			Popcorn:
			  Cheese
			  White cheddar cheese

Wise Choice		▽Butter popcorn	White cheddar popcorn

▽ Low sodium, 140 mg. or less per serving.

Popping Corn (Plain or Microwave)

ACCEPTABLE

■ **Without added fat or contains 1 gram or less fat per 3 cup serving (may be partially hydrogenated)**
These popping corns are preferred choices because they contain the least amount of fat. Use an air popper or a microwave popper to pop corn kernels without added fat.

■ **Reduced fat, 3 grams or less fat per 3 cup serving, contain acceptable partially hydrogenated oil or shortening**
These microwave popcorns are lower in fat than the ones in column three. Most contain less than 30% calories from fat.

■ **High fat, contain acceptable partially hydrogenated oils or shortening (LIMIT USE)**
Although these popping corns contain added acceptable fats, they are substantially higher in fat (approximately 50% fat). Limited intake is recommended.

NOT RECOMMENDED

■ **With added saturated fat**
Popping corn with added saturated fat is not recommended.

NOTE

■ The sodium content of popcorn varies depending on added salt. Unsalted popcorns contain 0-5 mg. per 3 cup serving. Salted popcorns may contain as much as 300 mg. per 3 cup serving. Sodium symbols are used to indicate high (▲) or low (▽) sodium **only** when sodium content is provided on the product label. Those products that are not identified with either symbol may be either high or low sodium or contain between 141-399 mg. sodium per serving.

BRAND	ACCEPTABLE			NOT RECOMMENDED
	Without added fat or contain 1 gram or less fat per 3 cup serving (may be partially hydrogenated)	Reduced fat, 3 grams or less fat per 3 cup serving, contain acceptable partially hydrogenated oil or shortening	High fat, contain acceptable partially hydrogenated oil or shortening (LIMIT USE)	With added saturated fat
Bascom's	Fancy colored popcorn			
Betty Crocker		Betty Crocker Pop-Secret microwave popcorn: ▽Light butter flavor	Betty Crocker Pop-Secret microwave popcorn: Butter flavor Light natural flavor Natural flavor	
Black Jewell	*Black Jewell popcorn*			
Bonnie Lee	▽Bonnie Lee popcorn			
Golden Valley Microwave Foods, Inc.		Act II Lite microwave popcorn: ★Natural	Act II Microwave popcorn: ★Natural	Act II Lite Microwave popcorn: Butter Act II Microwave popcorn: Butter Cheddar cheese
Jiffy Pop			★Microwave butter flavor popcorn	Jiffy Pop popcorn: Butter flavor
Kroger			Kroger microwave popcorn: Butter flavor Natural flavor	
Newman's Own			Newman's Own oldstyle picture show popcorn: All natural flavor Butter flavor	

▽ Low sodium, 140 mg. or less per serving.
★ High fiber, 3 g. or greater per serving.

BRAND	ACCEPTABLE			NOT RECOMMENDED
	Without added fat or contain 1 gram or less fat per 3 cup serving (may be partially hydrogenated)	Reduced fat, 3 grams or less fat per 3 cup serving, contain acceptable partially hydrogenated oil or shortening	High fat, contain acceptable partially hydrogenated oil or shortening (LIMIT USE)	With added saturated fat
Old Capital	Old Capital Ken Kercheval's popcorn			Microwave popcorn: *Natural flavor*
Orville Redenbacher	Orville Redenbacher's gourmet popcorn: ▽Original ▽White Orville Redenbacher's light gourmet microwave popcorn: ▽Butter flavored ▽Natural		Orville Redenbacher's gourmet microwave popcorn: ▽Butter flavor ▽Butter flavor, salt free *Light butter flavor* Natural Natural flavor, salt free	Orville Redenbacher's gourmet microwave popcorn: *Butter toffee* Caramel Cheddar cheese
Weight Watchers	▽Weight Watchers microwave popcorn			

▽ Low sodium, 140 mg. or less per serving.

SOUPS

Soups provide an excellent means of satisfying the appetite with few calories. Whether elegant or simple, soup also provides a means to incorporate wholesome vegetables, grains and legumes into the diet.

Commercially prepared soups are nutritious but can provide substantial amounts of sodium. Look for low sodium soups identified by a (▽) symbol for a healthier alternative.

Soups

ACCEPTABLE

■ **Without added fat**
These soups are preferred because they do not contain added fat.

▨ **With added unsaturated oil,** and

▨ **With added acceptable partially hydrogenated oil**
Soups in this and the preceding category contain added acceptable fats but for the most part, are relatively low in fat.

NOT RECOMMENDED

■ **With added saturated fat**
Soups with added saturated fat are not recommended. Soups listed in this column and marked with a (†) symbol have added saturated fat in the form of poultry or beef fat. These soups can be made acceptable by storing them in the refrigerator, allowing the fat to harden, and then skimming off the fat before reheating.

NOTE

■ Soups that contain unspecified vegetable oils should be avoided because the source of the oil is unknown.

■ Those soups marked with a (•) symbol contain egg yolks, usually as an ingredient in egg noodles. The amount of cholesterol per serving is small and should not be of concern for those following a low cholesterol diet.

■ Most soups are high in sodium. Sodium content varies widely depending on the amount of salt added. Unsalted soups can contain as little as 25 mg. sodium per 8 ounce serving, whereas regular soups average approximately 800-1000 mg. sodium per 8 ounce serving. Sodium symbols are used to indicate high (▲) or low (▽) sodium **only** when sodium content is provided on the product label. Those products that are not identified with either symbol may be either high or low sodium or contain between 141-399 mg. sodium per serving.

BRAND	ACCEPTABLE			NOT RECOMMENDED
	Without added fat	With added unsaturated oil	With added acceptable partially hydrogenated oil	With added saturated fat
Bascom's	Minestrone soup mix			
Baxter	Onion soup			Bean and mixed pepper vegetarian recipe soup Country garden vegetarian recipe Cream of asparagus Lobster bisque Vichyssoise
Borden	Chili starter New England style chowder starter		Beef vegetable soup starter •Chicken noodle soup starter Hearty beef stew starter	
Campbell's	Condensed: ▲Beef broth (bouillon) ▲Chicken gumbo ▲Consomme (beef) ▲Manhandler chili beef with beans ▲Manhandler vegetable beef ▲Zesty tomato Home Cookin' soup: ▲Bean and ham ▲Country vegetable ▲Hearty beef		Chunky soup: ▲•Chicken nuggets with vegetables and noodles ▲★*Homestyle bean* ▲Old fashioned chicken ▲*Tomato* ▲Vegetable ▲*Vegetarian vegetable* Condensed: ▲•Chicken noodle	Campbell's Cup: ▲•†Chicken noodle with white meat ▲•†Noodle soup with chicken broth *Tomato* Vegetable beef Chunky soup: Beef with country vegetables Chicken corn chowder ▲•†Chicken noodle with mushrooms

▲ High sodium, 400 mg. or greater per serving.

★ High fiber, 3 g. or greater per serving.

• Contains egg yolks.

† Some soups are listed in the "NOT RECOMMENDED" column simply because they have added poultry or beef fat. Broth based soups can be made acceptable if they are stored in the refrigerator allowing the fat to harden and then skimmed before heating.

BRAND	ACCEPTABLE			NOT RECOMMENDED
	Without added fat	With added unsaturated oil	With added acceptable partially hydrogenated oil	With added saturated fat
Campbell's (Cont'd)	Home Cookin' soup (Cont'd): ▲Split pea with ham Microwavable Campbell's Cup: Chili beef Quality soup mix: ▲•*Chicken noodle* Special Request: ▲Vegetable beef		Condensed (Cont'd): ▲Clam Chowder, Manhattan style ▲Clam chowder, New England style ▲★Homestyle bean ▲•Homestyle chicken noodle ▲Tomato ▲Vegetarian vegetable Condensed soup/dip: ▲★*Black bean* Special Request: ▲•Chicken noodle ▲Tomato soup	Chunky soup (Cont'd): ▲†Chicken rice ▲†Chicken vegetable Chili beef Creamy chicken with mushrooms *Creamy onion* Creole-style red beans and rice with sausage New England clam chowder Old fashioned bean and ham Old fashioned vegetable beef Pepper steak ▲†Sirloin burger Split pea and ham ▲†Turkey vegetable Condensed: Cheddar cheese Chicken 'n Dumplings ▲†Chicken and stars ▲†Chicken broth ▲•†Chicken noodle O's ▲•†Chicken vegetable

▲ High sodium, 400 mg. or greater per serving.
★ High fiber, 3 g. or greater per serving.
• Contains egg yolks.
† Some soups are listed in the "NOT RECOMMENDED" column simply because they have added poultry or beef fat. Broth based soups can be made acceptable if they are stored in the refrigerator allowing the fat to harden and then skimmed before heating.

Brand	Acceptable			Not Recommended
	Without added fat	With added unsaturated oil	With added acceptable partially hydrogenated oil	With added saturated fat
Campbell's (Cont'd)				Condensed (Cont'd): ▲†Chicken with rice Cream of asparagus Cream of broccoli Cream of celery Cream of chicken Cream of mushroom Cream of potato Cream of shrimp Creamy chicken mushroom *Creamy natural broccoli* ▲•†Curly noodle with chicken French onion ▲†Golden mushroom Green pea Homestyle beef noodle Homestyle cream of potato Homestyle cream of tomato ▲†Homestyle vegetable ▲†Manhandler beef with vegetable and barley ▲†Manhandler minestrone ▲•†Manhandler noodles and ground beef

▲ High sodium, 400 mg. or greater per serving.
• Contains egg yolks.
† Some soups are listed in the "NOT RECOMMENDED" column simply because they have added poultry or beef fat. Broth based soups can be made acceptable if they are stored in the refrigerator allowing the fat to harden and then skimmed before heating.

BRAND	ACCEPTABLE			NOT RECOMMENDED
	Without added fat	With added unsaturated oil	With added acceptable partially hydrogenated oil	With added saturated fat
Campbell's (Cont'd)				Condensed (Cont'd): ▲†Manhandler Scotch broth Manhandler split pea with ham and bacon Manhandler with beans and bacon ▲†Meatball alphabet Nacho cheese Old fashioned tomato rice Old fashioned vegetable Oyster stew ▲†Turkey vegetable Vegetable with beef stock ▲•†Wonton Condensed soup/dip: Creamy onion Home Cookin' soup: ▲†Chicken rice ▲•†Chicken with broad egg noodles Minestrone ▲†Tomato garden *Vegetable beef* Microwavable Campbell's Cup: Bean with bacon and ham •†Beef noodle flavor

▲ High sodium, 400 mg. or greater per serving.
• Contains egg yolks.
† Some soups are listed in the "NOT RECOMMENDED" column simply because they have added poultry or beef fat. Broth based soups can be made acceptable if they are stored in the refrigerator allowing the fat to harden and then skimmed before heating.

BRAND	ACCEPTABLE			NOT RECOMMENDED
	Without added fat	With added unsaturated oil	With added acceptable partially hydrogenated oil	With added saturated fat
Campbell's (Cont'd)				Microwavable Campbell's Cup (Cont'd): Chicken noodle •†Chicken noodle flavor †Chicken with rice ▲•†Noodle soup with chicken broth †Vegetable beef Quality soup mix: ▲†*Chicken rice Hearty noodle* ▲•†Noodle soup Onion Ready to serve, low sodium: ▽•†Chicken with noodles Chunky vegetable beef Split pea Tomato with tomato pieces Vegetable soup with beef stock Special Request: Bean with bacon ▲†Chicken with rice Cream of chicken Cream of mushroom Vegetable soup

▲ High sodium, 400 mg. or greater per serving.
▽ Low sodium, 140 mg. or less per serving.
• Contains egg yolks.
† Some soups are listed in the "NOT RECOMMENDED" column simply because they have added poultry or beef fat. Broth based soups can be made acceptable if they are stored in the refrigerator allowing the fat to harden and then skimmed before heating.

BRAND	ACCEPTABLE			NOT RECOMMENDED
	Without added fat	With added unsaturated oil	With added acceptable partially hydrogenated oil	With added saturated fat
Carmel Kosher		Soup base, chicken style		
College Inn			Beef broth	†Chicken broth
Crosse and Blackwell				*French style onion soup made with beef stock* Minestrone
Dominiques		Gazpacho: Ready to serve		Lentil sausage soup New England clam chowder Snapper turtle U.S. Senate bean *Watercress soup with mushrooms*

Edward and Sons	Instant miso cup:
	  Golden light soup
	  Rich, savory soup with seaweed			

El Rio	Chili no beans			

Estee	Low sodium, low calorie instant soup mix:
	  ▽Beef vegetable
	  ▽Cream of tomato
	  ▽Tomato
				Low sodium, low calorie instant soup mix:
				  ▽†Chicken noodle

Fantastic Foods		Fantastic noodles:
		  ▲Curry vegetable
				Fantastic noodles:
				  Creamy cheddar

▲ High sodium, 400 mg. or greater per serving.
▽ Low sodium, 140 mg. or less per serving.
† Some soups are listed in the "NOT RECOMMENDED" column simply because they have added poultry or beef fat. Broth based soups can be made acceptable if they are stored in the refrigerator allowing the fat to harden and then skimmed before heating.

BRAND	ACCEPTABLE			NOT RECOMMENDED
	Without added fat	With added unsaturated oil	With added acceptable partially hydrogenated oil	With added saturated fat
Fantastic Foods (Cont'd)		Fantastic noodles (Cont'd): ▲Miso vegetable ▲Tomato vegetable Vegetarian chili with beans		
Featherweight				Instant bouillon, no salt added: ▽†Beef flavor ▽†Chicken flavor
Hain	Hain Naturals: ▲•Chicken noodle soup Hain Naturals, no salt added: ▽Vegetable chicken soup Hain soup and recipe mix: ▲*Mushroom* ▲*Onion* Savory soup mix: ▲Minestrone ▲*Onion* ▲*Split pea* ▲*Vegetable*	Hain Naturals: ▲Italian vege-pasta ▲★Lentil ▲Minestrone ▲Vegetable chicken ▲Vegetarian vegetable Hain Naturals, low salt: ▽Vegetarian pasta Hain Naturals, no salt added: ▽Minestrone ▽Split-pea ▽★Vegetarian lentil ▽*Vegetarian vegetable*		Hain soup and recipe mix: Cheese and broccoli Hain soup and sauce mix: Cheese

▲ High sodium, 400 mg. or greater per serving.
▽ Low sodium, 140 mg. or less per serving.
★ High fiber, 3 g. or greater per serving.
• Contains egg yolks.
† Some soups are listed in the "NOT RECOMMENDED" column simply because they have added poultry or beef fat. Broth based soups can be made acceptable if they are stored in the refrigerator allowing the fat to harden and then skimmed before heating.

BRAND	ACCEPTABLE			NOT RECOMMENDED
	Without added fat	With added unsaturated oil	With added acceptable partially hydrogenated oil	With added saturated fat
Hain (Cont'd)		Hain soup and recipe mix: ▲Tomato Hain soup mix: ▲Vegetarian lentil		.
Harris Atlantic			Condensed soup: Oyster stew	Condensed soup: She-crab soup
Health Valley	No salt added soup: ▽Beef flavored broth ▽Chunky vegetable chicken ★Spicy vegetarian chili with beans	▲100% natural mushroom barley soup ★Black bean soup ★Chunky 5-bean vegetable soup ▲★Lentil soup ▽★Mild vegetarian chili with beans (no salt added) ★Mild vegetarian chili with beans ▲★Minestrone No salt added soup: ▽★Lentil soup ▽★Minestrone ▽★Potato leek ▽★Split pea		▲†Chicken broth No salt added soup: ▽†Chicken broth

▲ High sodium, 400 mg. or greater per serving.
▽ Low sodium, 140 mg. or less per serving.
★ High fiber, 3 g. or greater per serving.
† Some soups are listed in the "NOT RECOMMENDED" column simply because they have added poultry or beef fat. Broth based soups can be made acceptable if they are stored in the refrigerator allowing the fat to harden and then skimmed before heating.

BRAND	ACCEPTABLE			NOT RECOMMENDED
	Without added fat	With added unsaturated oil	With added acceptable partially hydrogenated oil	With added saturated fat
Health Valley (Cont'd)		No salt added soup (Cont'd): ▽Tomato ▽★Vegetable ▲Potato leek ▲Tomato ▲★Vegetable soup ▲★Vegetarian vegetable soup		
Herb-Ox				Bouillon cubes: †Beef †Chicken Instant bouillon: †Beef †Chicken Instant broth and seasoning: †Beef flavor †Chicken flavor ▽†Low sodium beef flavor ▽†Low sodium chicken flavor Onion Vegetable
Hodgson Mill	"Choice" 13 bean soup mix			

▲ High sodium, 400 mg. or greater per serving.
▽ Low sodium, 140 mg. or less per serving.
★ High fiber, 3 g. or greater per serving.
† Some soups are listed in the "NOT RECOMMENDED" column simply because they have added poultry or beef fat. Broth based soups can be made acceptable if they are stored in the refrigerator allowing the fat to harden and then skimmed before heating.

BRAND	ACCEPTABLE			NOT RECOMMENDED
	Without added fat	With added unsaturated oil	With added acceptable partially hydrogenated oil	With added saturated fat
Hormel				Microcup: ▲•†Hearty soup – chicken noodle Hearty soup – New England clam chowder
International Bazaar				Cream of asparagus *Cream of broccoli* Lobster bisque New England clam chowder Potato leek chowder
Knorr			Soup and recipe mix: ▲Asparagus ▲Cauliflower ▲Spinach ▲Tomato with basil ▲*Vegetable*	▲•†Chicken flavor noodle soup mix †Country barley soup mix Instant bouillon: †*Beef* †*Chicken* Instant soup: Cream of chicken flavor Instant soup mix: Chicken flavor noodle *Potato* Tomato Instant soup with croutons: *Cream of chicken* Cream of mushroom

▲ High sodium, 400 mg. or greater per serving.
• Contains egg yolks.
† Some soups are listed in the "NOT RECOMMENDED" column simply because they have added poultry or beef fat. Broth based soups can be made acceptable if they are stored in the refrigerator allowing the fat to harden and then skimmed before heating.

BRAND	ACCEPTABLE			NOT RECOMMENDED
	Without added fat	With added unsaturated oil	With added acceptable partially hydrogenated oil	With added saturated fat
Knorr (Cont'd)				Instant soup with croutons (Cont'd): *Cream of tomato* Cream of vegetable Soup and recipe mix: Fine herb ▲†French onion ▲†Leek Mushroom Soup mix: ▲•†Chicken flavor noodle
Kroger		Chunky soup: ▲Chunky vegetable ▲Chunky vegetable beef Condensed: ▲Tomato	Condensed: ▲Vegetarian vegetable Ramen Oriental noodle soup: ▲•Beef flavor ▲•Chicken flavor ▲•Shrimp flavor	Bouillon cubes: ▲†Beef ▲†Chicken Chunky soup: Chunky bean with ham Chunky beef with country vegetables ▲•†Chunky chicken soup Chunky clam chowder ▲†Chunky sirloin burger ▲†*Clear chicken broth* Condensed: Bean with bacon Chicken noodle ▲•†*Chicken O'Noodle*

▲ High sodium, 400 mg. or greater per serving.
• Contains egg yolks.
† Some soups are listed in the "NOT RECOMMENDED" column simply because they have added poultry or beef fat. Broth based soups can be made acceptable if they are stored in the refrigerator allowing the fat to harden and then skimmed before heating.

BRAND	ACCEPTABLE			NOT RECOMMENDED
	Without added fat	**With added unsaturated oil**	**With added acceptable partially hydrogenated oil**	**With added saturated fat**
Kroger (Cont'd)				Condensed (Cont'd): Cream of celery *Cream of chicken* Cream of mushroom Homestyle chicken noodle Vegetable beef Vegetable, made with beef stock Cream of potato
Lipton	Cup-a-soup Lite: •Lemon chicken		Cup-a-soup: ▲•Spring vegetable Lipton Recipe soup mix: ▲Onion ▲Onion-mushroom Lots-a-noodles: ▲Beef flavor	Cup-a-soup: Chicken noodle with white meat Green pea Tomato Cup-a-soup Creamy: Broccoli and cheese Cream of chicken Creamy broccoli Cup-a-soup Hearty: ▲•†Chicken and noodles Chicken supreme ▲•†Hearty chicken Cup-a-soup Lite: Golden creamy broccoli ▲†Oriental vegetable *Tomato and herb*

▲ High sodium, 400 mg. or greater per serving.
• Contains egg yolks.
† Some soups are listed in the "NOT RECOMMENDED" column simply because they have added poultry or beef fat. Broth based soups can be made acceptable if they are stored in the refrigerator allowing the fat to harden and then skimmed before heating.

BRAND	ACCEPTABLE			NOT RECOMMENDED
	Without added fat	With added unsaturated oil	With added acceptable partially hydrogenated oil	With added saturated fat
Lipton (Cont'd)				Lipton Hearty soup mix: ▲•†*Hearty chicken noodle* Hearty noodle Lots-a-noodles: ▲†Chicken flavor ▲†Oriental flavor ▲†Vegetable Soup mix: ▲•†Chicken noodle ▲•†Noodle soup
Lunch Bucket	Vegetable beef soup			▲•†Chicken noodle soup
Maggi			Bouillon cubes: Beef	Bouillon cubes: †Chicken
Morga				Vegetable bouillon cubes: Unsalted
Mrs. Grass			Soup and dip mix: Homestyle vegetable Onion Onion-mushroom	Soup mix: •†Homestyle chickeny flavored noodle •†Noodle soup
Mrs. Weiss				Soup mix: •†*Beef flavored kluski noodle soup* •†Chicken flavored old fashioned noodle soup

▲ High sodium, 400 mg. or greater per serving.
• Contains egg yolks.
† Some soups are listed in the "NOT RECOMMENDED" column simply because they have added poultry or beef fat. Broth based soups can be made acceptable if they are stored in the refrigerator allowing the fat to harden and then skimmed before heating.

BRAND	ACCEPTABLE			NOT RECOMMENDED
	Without added fat	With added unsaturated oil	With added acceptable partially hydrogenated oil	With added saturated fat
Mrs. Weiss (Cont'd)				Soup mix (Cont'd): •†Chicken kluski noodle soup
Nissin			Cup o' Noodle Oriental noodle soup: with Shrimp	Cup o' Noodle Oriental noodle soup: †Beef flavor †Chicken flavor †Chicken mushroom flavor
Panni			*Instant potato soup*	
Pepperidge Farm	*Borscht soup*		Black bean soup	"Shiitake" mushroom soup Bacon, lettuce and tomato Chicken curry soup Chicken with wild rice soup Corn chowder Cream of broccoli soup French onion Hunter's soup Lobster bisque New England clam chowder Oyster stew Vichyssoise Watercress
Pritikin	*Beef broth* Chicken broth (defatted)			

• Contains egg yolks.
† Some soups are listed in the "NOT RECOMMENDED" column simply because they have added poultry or beef fat. Broth based soups can be made acceptable if they are stored in the refrigerator allowing the fat to harden and then skimmed before heating.

BRAND	ACCEPTABLE			NOT RECOMMENDED
	Without added fat	With added unsaturated oil	With added acceptable partially hydrogenated oil	With added saturated fat
Pritikin (Cont'd)	*Chicken soup* Chicken soup with ribbon pasta ▽★Minestrone Vegetable			
Progresso	Chicken barley •Chicken noodle Chicken rice with vegetables Hearty chicken	Lentil Minestrone		†Beef barley •†Beef noodle †Beef vegetable Cream of chicken with mushrooms Cream of mushroom Green split pea New England clam chowder †Tomato beef with rotini †Vegetable
Rokeach		•Split pea and egg barley		
Stegner's				Mock turtle soup
Swanson				▲†Clear beef broth ▲†Clear chicken broth Natural Goodness with ⅓ less salt: ▲†Clear chicken broth
Sweet Sue				†Clear chicken broth

▲ High sodium, 400 mg. or greater per serving.
▽ Low sodium, 140 mg. or less per serving.
★ High fiber, 3 g. or greater per serving.
• Contains egg yolks.
† Some soups are listed in the "NOT RECOMMENDED" column simply because they have added poultry or beef fat. Broth based soups can be made acceptable if they are stored in the refrigerator allowing the fat to harden and then skimmed before heating.

BRAND	ACCEPTABLE			NOT RECOMMENDED
	Without added fat	**With added unsaturated oil**	**With added acceptable partially hydrogenated oil**	**With added saturated fat**
Tabatchnick	Frozen boil-in-bag soups: *Barley bean soup* •Minestrone		Frozen boil-in-bag soups: Barley mushroom Cabbage Lentil soup Pea soup Potato soup •Vegetable	Frozen boil-in-bag soups: Chicken broth with noodles and dumplings Cream of broccoli soup Cream of spinach
Telma				Beef flavor broth Consomme cube
Weight Watchers		▲Chunky vegetarian vegetable	•Chicken noodle Instant Broth 'n Seasoning mix: ▲Beef flavor	Cream of mushroom Instant Broth 'n Seasoning mix: ▲†Chicken flavor Turkey vegetable Vegetable with beef stock
Wyler's				Bouillon cubes: Beef flavor ▲†Chicken flavor

▲ High sodium, 400 mg. or greater per serving.
• Contains egg yolks.
† Some soups are listed in the "NOT RECOMMENDED" column simply because they have added poultry or beef fat. Broth based soups can be made acceptable if they are stored in the refrigerator allowing the fat to harden and then skimmed before heating.

References

1. Department of Health and Human Services: *The Surgeon General's Report on Nutrition and Health*. Washington, D.C., U.S. Government Printing Office, 1988 (DHHS Publication [PH 588-50210]).

2. Connor W.E., Connor S.L.: The Key Role of Nutritional Factors in the Prevention of Coronary Heart Disease. *Prev Med 1* (1):49-83, 1972.

3. National Academy of Sciences, Institute of Medicine, Food and Nutrition Board, Committee on the Nutrition Components of Food Labeling: *Nutrition Labeling Issues and Directions for the 1990's*. National Academy Press, Washington, D.C., 1990.

4. Keys A., Anderson J.T., Grande F.: Prediction of serum cholesterol responses of man to changes in fats in the diet. *Lancet* 2:959-966, 1957.

5. Hegstead D.M., McGandy R.B., Myers M.L., Stare F.J.: Quantitative effects of dietary fat on serum cholesterol in man. *Am J Clin Nutr* 17:281-295, 1965.

6. W. Kannel: Cholesterol in the Prediction of Atherosclerotic Disease. *Ann Intern Med* 90:85-91, 1979.

7. Halgrer, Levin, Rossner, Vessby Ledo: *Diet and Prevention of Coronary Heart Disease and Cancer*, 4th International Bergelius Symposium New York. Raven Press, 1986.

8. Report of the National Cholesterol Education Panel Program Expert Panel on detection, evaluation and treatment of high blood cholesterol in adults. *Arch Intern Med* 148:36-69, 1988.

9. Pooling Project Research Group: Relationship of blood pressure, serum cholesterol, smoking habit, relative weight and ECG abnormalities to incidence of major coronary events: final report of the pooling project. *J Chronic Dis* 31:201-212, 1978.

10. Castelli W.P.: Cholesterol and Lipids in the Risk of Coronary Artery Disease: The Framingham Heart Study. *Can J Cardiol* (supplement A):5A-10A, July 1988.

11. Anderson J.W.: Dietary fiber, lipids and atherosclerosis. *Am J Cardiol* 60:17G-22G, 1987.

12. Lipid Research Clinics Program. The Lipid Research Clinics Coronary Primary Prevention Trial results: II. The relationship of reduction in incidence of coronary heart disease to cholesterol lowering. *JAMA* 251:365-374, 1984.

13. Castelli W.P., Garrison R.J., Wilson P.W. et. al.: Incidence of Coronary Heart Disease and Lipoprotein Cholesterol Levels: The Framingham Study. *JAMA* 256(20):2835-2838, 1986.

14. Gordon D.J., Probstfield J.L., Garrison R.J. et. al.: High-density lipoprotein cholesterol and cardiovascular disease. Four prospective American studies. *Circulation* 79:8-15, 1989.

15. Burr M.L., Butland B.K.: Heart disease in British Vegetarians. *Am J Clin Nutr* 48:830-832, 1988.

16. Sacks F.M., Castelli W.P., Donner A., et. al.: Plasma lipids and lipoproteins in vegetarians and controls. *N Eng J Med* 292:1148-1151, 1975.

17. Frick M.H., Elo O., Haapa, K.A., et. al.: Helsinki Heart Study Primary Prevention Trial with genfibrozil in middle-aged men with dyslipidemia. *N Engl J Med* 317:1237-1245, 1987.

18. Egusa G., Beltz W.F., Grundy S.M., Howard B.V.: The influence of obesity on the metabolism of apolipoprotein B in man. *J Clin Invest* 76:596-603, 1985.

19. Keys A., Anderson J.T., Grande F.: Serum cholesterol response to changes in the diet. IV. Particular saturated fatty acids in the diet. *Metabolism* 14:776-787, 1965.

20. Mattson, F.H., Grundy S.M.: Comparison of effects of dietary saturated, monounsaturated, and polyunsaturated fatty acids on plasma lipids and lipoproteins. *J Lipid Res* 26:194-202, 1985.

21. Keys A., ed.: Coronary heart disease in seven countries. *Circulation* 41(suppl):I-1, 1970.

22. Grundy S.M.: Comparison of monounsaturated fatty acids and carbohydrates for lowering plasma cholesterol. *N Engl J Med* 314:745-748, 1986.

23. Grundy S.M., Florentin L., Nix D., et. al.: Comparison of monounsaturated fatty acids and carbohydrates for reducing raised levels of plasma cholesterol in man. *Am J Clin Nutr* 47:965-969, 1988.

24. Grundy S.M.: Monounsaturated fatty acids, plasma cholesterol and coronary heart disease. *Am J Clin Nutr* 45:1168-1175, 1987.

25. Vega G.L., Groszek E., Wolf R., Grundy S.M.: Influence of polyunsaturated fats on plasma lipoprotein composition and apolipoprotein. *J Lipid Res* 23:811-822, 1982.

26. Shepherd J., Packard C.J., Grundy S.M., et. al.: Effects of saturated and polyunsaturated fat diets on the chemical composition and metabolism of low-density lipoproteins in man. *J Lipid Res* 21:91-99, 1980.

27. Dreon D.M., Vranizan K.M., Krauss R.M., Austin M.A., Wood P.D.: The effects of polyunsaturated fat vs. monounsaturated fat on plasma lipoprotein. *JAMA* 263:2462-2466, 1990.

28. Parthasarathy S., Khoo J.C., Miller E. et. al.: Low density Lipoprotein rich in oleic acid is protected against oxidative modification: Implications for dietary prevention of atherosclerosis. *Proc Natl Acad Sci* 87:3894-3898, 1990.

29. National Academy of Science, National Research Council, Committee on Diet, Nutrition, and Cancer. *Diet, Nutrition, and Cancer.* Washington, D.C.: National Academy Press, 1982.

30. Bananome A., Grundy S.M.: Effects of dietary stearic acid on plasma cholesterol and lipoprotein levels. *N Eng J Med* 318:1244-1248, 1988.

31. Mensink R.P., Katan M.B.: Effect of Dietary Trans-Fatty Acids on High-Density and Low-Density Lipoprotein Cholesterol Levels In Healthy Subjects. *N Engl J Med* 323(7):439-445, 1990.

32. United States Department of Agriculture, Agriculture Handbook No. 8-4: *Composition of Foods: Fats and Oils — Raw, Processed, and Prepared.* Washington, D.C., U.S. Government Printing Office, 1979.

33. Committee on Nutrition, American Heart Association: *Dietary Guidelines for Healthy American Adults: A Statement for Physicians and Health Professionals.* 1986.

34. Anderson J.W., Story L., Sieling B., et. al.: Hypocholesterolemic effects of oat bran or bean intake for hypercholesterolemic men. *Am J Clin Nutr* 40:1146-1155, 1984.

35. Anderson J.W.: Health implications of wheat fiber. *Am J Clin Nutr* 41:1103-1112, 1985.

36. Anderson J.W.: High-fibre diets for diabetic and hypertriglyceridemic patients. *Can Med Assoc J* 123(10):975-979, 1980.

37. Karlstrom B., Vessby B., Asp N.G., Boberg M., Gustafsson I.B., Lithell H., and Werner I.: Effects of an increased content of cereal fiber in the diet of Type 2 (non-insulin-dependent) diabetic patients. *Diabetologia* 26:272-277, 1984.

38. Butrum R.R., Clifford C.K. and Lanza E.: NCI dietary guidelines: rationale. *Am J Cl Nutr* 48(3 Suppl):888-895, 1988.

39. Abraham S. and Carroll M.D.: *Fats, Cholesterol and Sodium Intake in the Diet of Persons 1-74 Years.* United States. Advance Data No. 54. U.S. Department of Health, Education, and Welfare, Washington, D.C. 1981.

40. Dahl L.K.: Possible role of salt intake in the development of essential hypertension Pp. 53-65 in P. Cottier and K.D. Bock, eds. *Essential Hypertension: An International Symposium.* Springer-Verlag, Heidelberg, Federal Republic of Germany, 1960.

41. Pennington J.A.T., Wilson D.B., Newell R.F., Hartland B.F., Johnson R.D. and Vanderveen J.E.: Selected minerals in food surveys, 1974 to 1981/82. *J Am Diet Assoc* 84:771-780, 1984.

42. National Research Council, Commission on Life Sciences, Food and Nutrition Board, Subcommittee on the Tenth Edition of the RDAs: *Recommended Dietary Allowances 10th Edition.* National Academy Press, Washington, D.C., 1989.

43. National Research Council, Report of the Committee on Diet and Health, Food and Nutrition Board: *Diet and Health: Implications for Reducing Chronic Disease Risk.* National Academy Press, Washington, D.C., 1989.

44. Thelle D.S., Arnesen E., Forde O.H.: The Tromso heart study: Does coffee raise serum cholesterol? *N Engl J Med* 308:1454-1457, 1983.

45. U.S. Department of Agriculture, U.S. Department of Health and Human Services. *Dietary Guidelines for Americans, 3RD edition.* U.S. GPO: 1990 — 273-930.

46. Kromhout D., Bosschieter E.B., Coulander C.: The inverse relationship between fish consumption and 20-year mortality from coronary heart disease. *N Engl J Med* 312:1205-1209, 1985.

APPENDICES

Appendix A

Status of Current Federal Policy for Selected Descriptors

Nutrient and Term	FDA Criteria	USDA Criteria
Calcium	No regulation; informal policy developed for trial shelf labeling programs[a]	No regulation
Source	At least 100 mg of calcium per serving	
Good source	At least 250 mg of calcium per serving	
Excellent source	At least 400 mg of calcium per serving	
Calories		
Low calorie	Less than or equal to 40 calories per serving and less than or equal to 0.4 calories/g (21 CFR § 105.66(c))	Less than or equal to 40 calories per serving and less than or equal to 0.4 calories/g (USDA, 1982a)
Reduced calorie	At least one-third fewer calories, but otherwise nutritionally equivalent to the food it replaces; requires a statement of comparison (21 CFR § 105.66(d))	At least a 25 percent reduction is required along with an explanatory statement and quantitative information (USDA, 1982a)
Sugar free No sugar	Must be low calorie, reduced calorie, have a comparative claim, or descriptor must be followed by a phrase indicating it is not a low calorie food (21 CFR § 105.66(f))	Negative claims are permitted if it is not clear from product name that the ingredient is not contained in the product (USDA, 1987a)
Cholesterol		
Cholesterol free No cholesterol	Tentative final rule; less than 2 mg of cholesterol per serving and 5 g or less of total fat per serving and 20 percent or less of total fat on a dry weight basis and 2 g or less of saturated fatty acids per serving and 6 percent or less of saturated fatty acids on a dry weight basis[b]	No such claims expected for meat products[c]

a Letter to J.S. Kahan and B.L. Rubin, Hogan and Hartson, Washington, D.C., by R.J. Ronk, Center for Food Safety and Applied Nutrition, Food and Drug Administration, DHHS, August 26, 1988.
b 55 Fed. Reg. 29,456 – 29,473 (July 19, 1990).
c S. Jones, Standards and Labeling Division, Food Safety and Inspection Service, USDA, personal communication, 1990.

Nutrient and Term	FDA Criteria	USDA Criteria
Cholesterol (Cont'd)		
Cholesterol free food	Tentative final rule; must meet conditions for free of cholesterol, cholesterol free, or no cholesterol and inherently contain less than 2 mg of cholesterol per serving without the benefit of special processing or reformulation to alter cholesterol content; provided that such labeling clearly refers to all foods of that type and not merely to the particular brand to which the labeling attaches[b]	No regulation (see low cholesterol meal)
Low cholesterol Low in cholesterol	Tentative final rule; less than or equal to 20 mg of cholesterol per serving and 0.2 mg or less of cholesterol per g of food, and 5 g or less of total fat per serving and 20 percent or less of total fat on a dry weight basis and 2 g or less of saturated fatty acids per serving and 6 percent or less of saturated fatty acids on a dry weight basis[b]	No regulation; tentatively using FDA's proposed definition[c]
Low cholesterol meal	No regulation	No regulation; working policy of no more than 20 mg/100 g of product[c]
Reduced cholesterol Cholesterol reduced	Tentative final rule; at least 75 percent reduction of cholesterol content compared with that in the food it resembles in organoleptic properties and for which it substitutes, provided that the label of such a food also bears clear and concise quantitative information comparing the product's per serving cholesterol content with that of the food it replaces[b]	No regulation; tentatively permitting comparative claims that are reduced at least 25 percent from the regular policy[c]

b 55 Fed. Reg. 29,456 – 29,473 (July 19, 1990).
c S. Jones, Standards and Labeling Division, Food Safety and Inspection Service, USDA, personal communication, 1990.

Nutrient and Term	FDA Criteria	USDA Criteria
Fat		
Lean	No regulation	May contain no more than 10 percent fat (except for ground beef and hamburger, which may contain a 25 percent reduction from standard of 30 percent fat — i.e., no more than 22.5 percent fat); brand names must meet standard or lower-fat definition except dinners/entrees designed for weight loss or maintenance, which must include abbreviated nutrition label (USDA, 1987b)
Extra lean	No regulation	May contain no more than 5 percent fat (except for ground beef and hamburger — the exception described above will also qualify for extra lean) (USDA, 1987b)
Low fat	No regulation; policy guideline states that less than or equal to 2 g of fat per serving and less than or equal to 10 percent fat on a dry weight basis[d]	May contain no more than 10 percent fat (USDA, 1987b)
Reduced fat Lower fat	No regulation; policy guideline states that at least 50 percent reduction from the regular product accompanied by a statement of comparison[d]	Comparative claims must have achieved at least a 25 percent reduction (or difference) in fat (or lean) (USDA, 1987b)
Fiber	No regulation; informal policy developed for trial shelf labeling programs[a]	No regulation[c]
Source	At least 2 g of fiber per serving	No regulation[c]

[a] Letter to J.S. Kahan and B.L. Rubin, Hogan and Hartson, Washington, D.C., by R.J. Ronk, Center for Food Safety and Applied Nutrition, Food and Drug Administration, DHHS, August 26, 1988.

[c] S. Jones, Standards and Labeling Division, Food Safety and Inspection Service, USDA, personal communication, 1990.

[d] Pennington, J.A.T., V.L. Wilkening, and J.E. Vanderveen. 1990. Descriptive terms for food labeling. J. Nutr. Ed. 22(1):51-54; and R.E. Newberry, Division of Regulatory Guidance, Center for Food Safety and Applied Nutrition, Food and Drug Administration, DHHS, personal communication, 1990.

Nutrient and Term	FDA Criteria	USDA Criteria
Fiber (Cont'd)		
Good source (FDA) Significant source (USDA)	At least 5 g of fiber per serving	No regulation; working policy of at least 3 g of fiber per serving[c]
Excellent source (FDA)	At least 8 g of fiber per serving	No regulation[c]
Fresh	May not be applied to foods that have been subjected to any form of heat or chemical processing (Compliance Policy Guide 7120.06)	May be used if not cured, canned, hermetically sealed, dried, or chemically preserved — not shelf stable; for poultry, cannot be used if frozen at or below 0°F; brand names exempt (USDA, 1989a)
Lite and Light	No regulation; working policy considers lite to mean reduced calorie, one-third fewer calories, unless defined elsewhere (i.e., a food standard, for example, light cream, or an obvious example, light versus heavy syrup)[e]	May refer to fat, salt, sodium, breading, and/or other components; a 25 percent reduction is required along with an explanatory statement and quantitative information; dinners/entrees designed for weight loss or maintenance must include abbreviated nutrition label (USDA, 1982a)
Natural	No regulation	May be used if product contains no artificial flavor, coloring, or chemical preservative and the product and its ingredients are not more than minimally processed, along with explanatory statement (USDA, 1982b)
Organic	No regulation	No regulation; not permitted
Sodium		
Sodium free	Less than 5 mg of sodium per serving (21 CFR § 101.13(a)(1))	Less than 5 mg of sodium per serving (USDA, 1984)

c S. Jones, Standards and Labeling Division, Food Safety and Inspection Service, USDA, personal communication, 1990.

e Letter to M.E. Thompson, Kraft, Inc., Glenview, IL, by S.A. Miller, Center for Food Safety and Applied Nutrition, Food and Drug Administration, DHHS, July 9, 1987; and R.E. Newberry, Division of Regulatory Guidance, Center for Food Safety and Applied Nutrition, Food and Drug Administration, DHHS, personal communication, 1990.

Nutrient and Term	FDA Criteria	USDA Criteria
Sodium (Cont'd)		
Very low sodium	Less than or equal to 35 mg of sodium per serving (21 CFR § 101.13(a)(2))	Less than or equal to 35 mg of sodium per serving (USDA, 1984)
Low sodium	Less than or equal to 140 mg of sodium per serving (21 CFR § 101.13(a)(3))	Less than or equal to 140 mg of sodium per serving (USDA, 1984)
Reduced sodium	At least 75 percent reduction of sodium compared with that in the food it replaces; also requires a statement of comparison; additional comparative claims are permitted if at least 25 percent sodium reduction is achieved and is accompanied by explanatory statement (21 CFR § 101.13(a)(4))	At least 75 percent reduction of sodium compared with that in the food it replaces; also requires a statement of comparison; additional comparative claims are permitted if at least 25 percent sodium reduction is achieved and is accompanied by explanatory statement (USDA, 1984)
. . . source of	No regulation; informal policy developed for shelf labeling programs[f]	No regulation; FDA's definitions used as basis for working policy[c]
Fair Significant	At least 10 percent or more of U.S. RDA per serving	
Good	At least 25 percent or more of U.S. RDA per serving	
Excellent	At least 40 percent or more of U.S. RDA per serving	

c S. Jones, Standards and Labeling Division, Food Safety and Inspection Service, USDA, personal communication, 1990.
f Letter to O. Matthews, Giant Food, Inc., Washington, D.C., by Sanford A. Miller, Center for Food Safety and Applied Nutrition, Food and Drug Administration, DHHS, July 16, 1986.

INDEX

GROCERY SHOPPING GUIDE and HIGH FIT – LOW FAT ORDER FORM

Make check payable to:
The University of Michigan Press

Mail to:
The University of Michigan Press
P.O. Box 1104
Ann Arbor, MI 48106

☐ Please send me ____ copies of the **Grocery Shopping Guide** $18.95 each _____
☐ Please send me ____ copies of the **High Fit – Low Fat Cookbook** $14.95 each _____

Michigan Residents, add 4% sales tax _____
+ $1.00 shipping & handling (for 1st book only) _____
+ $ .25 shipping & handling for each additional book _____
TOTAL _____

Name _____
Address _____
City _____
State _____ Zip _____
Daytime Phone _____

Deliver to: (if different address)
Name _____
Address _____
City _____
State _____ Zip _____

My payment is by:
☐ Check   ☐ Money Order   ☐ VISA   ☐ MasterCard

Credit Card Number (all digits) _____
Expiration Date _____

Signature: _____
(required if using credit card)

Order Form